Innovations
in Health Care Delivery

*Stephen S. Mick
and Associates*

Innovations in Health Care Delivery

Insights for Organization Theory

 Jossey-Bass Publishers

San Francisco • Oxford • 1990

INNOVATIONS IN HEALTH CARE DELIVERY
Insights for Organization Theory
by Stephen S. Mick and Associates

Copyright © 1990 by: Jossey-Bass Inc., Publishers
350 Sansome Street
San Francisco, California 94104
&
Jossey-Bass Limited
Headington Hill Hall
Oxford OX3 0BW

Library of Congress Cataloging-in-Publication Data
Mick, Stephen S.
    Innovations in health care delivery : insights for organization
theory / Stephen S. Mick and associates.—1st ed.
        p.   cm—(The Jossey-Bass health series)
    Includes bibliographacial references.
    Includes Index.
    ISBN 1-55542-281-0
    1. Health services administration—United States.   2. Medical
care—United States—Planning.   I. Title   II. Series
    [DNLM: 1. Delivery of Health Care—organization & administration—
United States.   2. Health Planning—United States.   3. Technology,
Medical.   W 84 AA1   M56i]
RA971.M484   1990
362.1'0973—dc20   90-4840
DNLM/DLC   CIP
for Library of Congress

Manufactured in the United States of America

The paper in this book meets the guidelines for
permanence and durability of the Committee on
Production Guidelines for Book Longevity of the
Council on Library Resources.

JACKET DESIGN BY WILLI BAUM

Nwst
/AEC 9890

FIRST EDITION

Code 9075

The Jossey-Bass Health Series

Contents

Preface

Innovations in Health Care Delivery describes and evaluates some new and revised approaches to organization theory. As we witnessed unusual environmental change in health care in the 1980s, many of us were struck by the ability of some health care organizations to make creative responses to the opportunities change provided while other organizations seemed powerless before the same environmental shifts. The contributors to this book, like others before us, became dissatisfied with the inability of existing theoretical paradigms to explain these different responses. And so we sought fresh ways to unravel riddles of organizational life in health care. Thus, we challenge conventional ideas, reified by decades of relatively stable organizational arrangements within relatively placid environments, and some we even abandon.

Within this broad context, the charge to each group of authors was to present new thinking about a topic of their choice. I made no further effort to direct or dictate what was to be written, to supply a narrow motif around which all the chapters had to revolve, or to develop a single, integrated theme. Books edited in that way have their place to be sure. But the aim here was to present diverse views on what the turmoil in the health care environment of the 1980s implied for organization theory.

Although the chapters that follow do not bridge all the gaps between current empirical complexity and theoretical descriptions and explanations, they do represent creative and flexible thinking about the status of organization theory in health care. The contrib-

utors address some issues in health care organization theory without
the usual, often stultifying, constraints that are self-imposed by disciplinary training or externally imposed by the canons of journal
publication. The result is, I believe, an unusual collection of chapters that shed light on a sector rife with change and at the same time
provide insight into organization theory generally.

The open and general charge to the contributors does not
mean, however, that convergences do not exist. Several crosscutting
themes emerged: environmental complexity and interpenetration,
organizational innovation, strategic management activity, and economic approaches to organization theory. These themes correspond, not without coincidence, with several key concerns: cost
containment and efficiency; shifts to public and private incentives
that favor mergers, diversification, corporate restructuring, and a
broadened conception of organizational arrangements; appeals to
business technique and logic; and the rise in importance of strategic
planning.

The Book's Challenge

Many people in classrooms, seminars, and professional meetings
have found themselves at a loss in attempting to fit a refractory
empirical reality into time-honored models. Hence, in writing this
book, we have sought some new approaches and answers. Our book
is one of the very few that takes a searching look at the status of and
change in organization theory in health care. At an empirical level,
we ask questions that have immediate policy and managerial im-
port: Is the conflict between professionals and organizations as
dichotomous as we have generally depicted it to be? Are hospitals
helpless entities, caught in a web of constituents' conflicting values
and demands and dependent on federal and other public largesse,
unable to adapt and doomed to failure? Are the activities of profit-
seeking organizations antithetical to the larger goals of a service
sector designed to perform one of the most personal and consequen-
tial of human activities—caring for the ill? Are hospital administrators who act conservatively, well within the bounds of careful
cost accounting, the ones who will ensure the survival of their institutions? Or are the risk takers in the ascendancy?

Questions such as these lead us to ask others that are more theoretical: What new or different typologies capture the novel organizational arrangements that emerged in the 1980s? How can we understand and explain the apparent loss in a single decade of the authority that medical professionals held for much of the twentieth century? What models explain and predict the expansion of hospitals into certain service areas and their simultaneous contraction in others? Can existing theory describe and explain innovation in health care organizations as well as their adoption of new technology? Is the interest in strategic management and planning simply a form of futurism, or educated guesswork, about which activities health care organizations should undertake? Or is it a perspective that fruitfully reinvigorates in organization theory notions of voluntaristic discretion—in contradiction to theoretical positions subordinating the role of managerial action to the power of markets and impersonal social forces? This level of questioning characterizes the chapters in this book.

Overview of the Contents

Although the chapters may be read in any order, as each one is complete in its own right, the chapter arrangement is in a sequence that emphasizes a progression of themes and ideas. These themes include, first, the complexity and density of organizational environments in health care; second, organizational innovation; third, strategic activity; and, fourth, economic approaches to organization theory.

Chapter One is an overview of the changes and their causes in the health care environment of the 1980s. This background discussion merges into a presentation of the above-mentioned themes and convergences of the chapters in this book and of the research avenues they suggest.

In Chapter Two, W. Richard Scott and Elaine V. Backman document the influence that the study of occupations, particularly of the profession of medicine, has had on the development of health care organization theory. They demonstrate how the field is focusing less on medical professionals so that the impact on organizations of other forces, such as the state, can be clearly seen and studied. Scott and Backman emphasize the growth and explanatory potential of institutional theory, and they suggest that institutional theory, with its concern with organizational adaptation to environmental forces, sheds new light on ethical issues in health care.

While Scott and Backman provide an appreciation for the terminology and explanatory power of institutional theory, Jeffrey A. Alexander and Thomas A. D'Aunno, in Chapter Three, take institutional theory a step further. By focusing on three questions— From what institutional environment has the health care sector evolved? How is the institutional environment changing? What impact might this change have on health care organizations?—Alexander and D'Aunno propose a way for institutional theory to be strengthened and refined.

Chapter Four, by Arnold D. Kaluzny, Joseph P. Morrissey, and Martha M. McKinney, addresses the emergence of a new organizational form in health care: Community Clinical Oncology Programs (CCOPs), the organizational products of a federally funded research effort to diffuse cancer-treatment and cancer-control information to patients and providers across the nation. The authors hypothesize that the increasing density of interorganizational networks and multileveled administrative systems, as well as the quickening pace of technological innovation, demand new approaches to describe and explain the organizational arrangements that emerge.

James W. Begun, Roice D. Luke, and Dennis D. Pointer make the point in Chapter Five that out of the complex matrix of interorganizational relations arise new relationships between physicians and hospitals. They argue that a new taxonomic scheme based on organizational strategy and structure is required to capture the characteristics of these relationships, and they show the implication of these new relationships for managerial practice as well as new research avenues.

Strategy, introduced by Begun and his associates, takes center stage in Chapter 6. Stephen M. Shortell and Edward J. Zajac review the rise in importance of strategic thinking among health care managers and the contributions to date of health care analysts to strategic management theory. Focusing on strategic change and adaptation as well as on alliance building, they present a systematic research agenda for theory development as it emerges from the situation in health care.

Chapter Seven, by Laura Roper Renshaw, John R. Kimberly, and J. Sanford Schwartz, uses the case of magnetic resonance imaging (MRI) technology to illustrate the need for new and hybrid approaches to explain the often unconventional patterns of technology diffusion in the health care sector. The authors highlight the role of private venture capital and entrepreneurs, and they propose a unique adaptation of population ecology theory to capture features of environmental support and managerial strategy, both powerful forces in the spread of MRIs.

In Chapter Eight, I introduce another theme in this book: the application of transaction-cost economics to organization theory through a focus on vertical integration, a widespread phenomenon in health care in the 1980s. I observe that the transaction-cost market-failure paradigm (that organizational control is an efficient solution to the exchange of services when market exchange mechanisms break down) is at odds with recent strategic management theory and that a synthesis of the two approaches is required if any answer is to be found to the question of why health care organizations integrate vertically.

Transaction-cost economics receives central treatment in Chapter Nine. The movement toward integrated health care systems, including managed health care programs, is described by Robert E. Hurley and Mary L. Fennell, who assert that organization theory has not provided much insight into this phenomenon. They hypothesize that transaction-cost economics is applicable to managed care in Medicaid programs and mental health services.

Audience

Academics and students, both inside and outside health care, will find *Innovations in Health Care Delivery* of interest. Managers, health care practitioners, physicians and clinicians who have managerial roles, and others who seek to understand the diverse options available to them in changing environments will find the book helpful: Several chapters point out managerial issues associated with organizational change and adaptation. Also, policy analysts will find that the book provides different insights into the reactions of organizations to explicit and implicit policies devised during the 1980s.

Acknowledgments

I wish to thank the editors at Jossey-Bass for their encouragement and support in all stages of writing and assembling this book. Their continuing enthusiasm has kept the momentum going. In particular, thanks are due to Alis Valencia, who helped me envision this undertaking, and to Rebecca L. McGovern, who inspected the piles of manuscripts that I sent her, managed the editorial process, and offered advice on numerous points, all with grace and good humor. Xenia Lisanevich was very helpful in straightening out the final details. All the authors thank Martin P. Charns, Duncan Neuhauser, and an anonymous reviewer for their remarkably thorough and conscientious critiques. The organization and structure of the book are my own responsibility. My principal hope is that my colleagues and I have been successful in provoking comment and discussion and that the field will be better for it.

Ann Arbor, Michigan   Stephen S. Mick
June 1990

The Authors

Stephen S. Mick is associate professor in the Department of Health Services Management and Policy, School of Public Health, University of Michigan. He received his B.A. degree (1965) from Stanford University in psychology and his Ph.D. degree (1973) from Yale University in sociology. Mick taught sociology at Middlebury College; he also taught public health and health care organization and management at Yale University, Oklahoma University, the University of Washington, Johns Hopkins University, and the University of Michigan.

Mick's research focuses on a variety of areas in health services research and organizational analysis. His published work includes a book, *The Alien Doctors: Foreign Medical Graduates in American Hospitals* (1978, with R. A. Stevens and L. W. Goodman), and numerous journal articles on the subjects of health manpower, general medical care, and organization and management.

Jeffrey A. Alexander is associate professor in the Department of Health Services Management and Policy, School of Public Health, University of Michigan.

Elaine V. Backman is assistant professor in the Department of Sociology, Harvard University.

James W. Begun is professor in the Department of Health Administration, Medical College of Virginia, Virginia Commonwealth University.

Thomas A. D'Aunno is assistant professor in the Department of Health Services Management and Policy, School of Public Health, University of Michigan.

Mary L. Fennell is professor of sociology, Pennsylvania State University.

Robert E. Hurley is assistant professor in the Department of Health Administration, Medical College of Virginia, Virginia Commonwealth University.

Arnold D. Kaluzny is professor in the Department of Health Policy and Administration, School of Public Health, University of North Carolina, Chapel Hill. He is also a research associate at the Health Services Research Center at the university and a member of the university's Lineberger Cancer Center.

John R. Kimberly is professor in the Department of Management, The Wharton School, University of Pennsylvania.

Roice D. Luke is professor in and chairman of the Department of Health Administration, Medical College of Virginia, Virginia Commonwealth University.

Martha M. McKinney is research assistant at the Health Services Research Center, University of North Carolina, Chapel Hill. She is also Cancer Prevention Fellow at the National Cancer Institute.

Joseph P. Morrissey is associate professor in the Department of Social and Administrative Medicine, School of Medicine, University of North Carolina, Chapel Hill. He is also associate director of the university's Health Services Research Center.

Dennis D. Pointer is Arthur Graham Glasgow Professor in the Department of Health Administration, Medical College of Virginia, Virginia Commonwealth University.

Laura Roper Renshaw is grant manager for Oxfam America.

J. Sanford Schwartz is associate professor of medicine and health care systems; Robert D. Eilers Associate Professor of Health Management and Economics; senior scholar in clinical epidemiology, School of Medicine and Wharton School of Business; and executive director of the Leonard Davis Institute of Health Economics, University of Pennsylvania.

W. Richard Scott is professor in the Department of Sociology, Stanford University.

Stephen M. Shortell is A. C. Buehler Distinguished Professor of Hospital and Health Services Management and professor of organization behavior, J. L. Kellogg Graduate School of Management, Northwestern University.

Edward J. Zajac is assistant professor of organization behavior, J. L. Kellogg Graduate School of Management, Northwestern University.

Innovations
in Health Care Delivery

1

Themes, Issues, and Research Avenues

Stephen S. Mick

The chapters in this book are original efforts to help advance the field of organization theory. Specifically, this book aims to demonstrate the contribution that analysts of health care organizations can make to an understanding of organizations generally. Each author uses the health care sector and its constituent organizations as a prism to shed light on some current issues and debates in the broader field. Therefore, the book maintains a tradition of health care analysts' informing organization theory. I should point out that I am not arguing that health care organizations are unique. This issue continues to be debated, and Kimberly (1985) and Shortell and Kaluzny (1988), among others, present various perspectives on it. My view is that scholars who spend most of their time on a particular phenomenon are more likely than those who do not to appreciate its intricacies, nuances, and evolution. Their capacity to see the contribution of their studies to a larger relevant field may, therefore, be significant. Such may be the case with those of us committed to the study of health care. That health care organizations may be "special" is not the point; that we might see more in them than others is.

There is nothing new about the use of health care organizations to develop, illuminate, or expand organization theory. Examples abound and include work such as Fox's (1959) account of physician/patient relations surrounding experimental medicine in a hospital setting, Perrow's (1961) work on organizational goals, the papers by Levine and White (1961) and by Levine, White, and Paul

1

(1963) on exchange and cooperation among community health agencies, Goffman's (1961) classic study of mental hospitals, Duff and Hollingshead's (1968) analysis of quality of care and internal hospital stratification, Freidson's (1975) study of professional control in an organizational setting, Milner's (1980) monograph on symbiotic relations among hospitals, and much more. Testimony to this contribution of analysts of health care organizations to organization theory can be found in the detailed reviews of Croog and Ver Steeg (1972), Levine and White (1972), and Georgopoulos (1975).

These authors studied different problems in the health care sector, learned from them, and helped enrich our comprehension of health care as well as non-health care organizations. Our efforts here are no different in intent and, we hope, no less capable of directing inquiry into new areas. Those of us who study health care and its organizations have, by the events of the 1980s, been challenged to revise our vision of what organizations are and how they interact with their environments.

Environmental Changes in Health Care

Characteristics of the health care environment of the 1980s caused many of us to be puzzled by what we saw. These characteristics included the addition of nonlocal and multilayered authority structures to and sometimes their replacement of conventional physician/administrator/governing board structures; the convergence of hospital structures, goals, and performance regardless of for-profit or not-for-profit, religious or secular status; and the addition of diversified services only remotely related to the provision of health care.

For example, surgeons in hundreds of freestanding outpatient surgical centers around the nation performed procedures once considered impossible to do outside the concrete confines of acute-care hospitals. New and innovative organizational arrangements sprang up, some of them strange, defying easy description. Here one can cite the growth of third-party administrators, whose role was (and is) mainly to effect complicated contractual relations among employers, employees, insurers, and delivery organizations for a vast array of health care "products." Or one can cite hospital systems, both for-profit and not-for-profit, that have amassed vast resources for striking new construction, modernization, and diversification.

As a final example, there are the preferred provider organizations (PPOs), almost entirely new to the 1980s, although some would consider health maintenance organizations (HMOs) and their precursors, prepaid group practices, as historical antecedents. PPOs offer various health services delivered by specified physicians and hospitals at reduced costs for specified groups of enrollees. They generally have the following characteristics: a limited number of physicians and hospitals, negotiated fee schedules, utilization management (controls on the appropriateness and volume of clinical services), and consumer choice of provider with incentives to use the PPO providers (de Lissovoy, Rice, Ermann, and Gabel, 1986). Additionally, PPOs frequently offer rapid claims reporting, monitoring, and settlement, and they engage in flexible and timely market-driven behavior (underbidding traditional health insurers for a new client's business). Enrollees are not required to use the PPO physicians or hospitals. They do not forfeit their health-insurance coverage if they use out-of-plan providers, although they usually have to pay additional fees if they do so. Such freedom of choice distinguishes PPOs from HMOs because HMOs typically do not reimburse those who use an out-of-plan provider. (Even this restriction in HMOs is beginning to change; see Feldman, Kralewski, and Dowd, 1989.) Hence, PPOs are thought to be midway between the extremes of fee-for-service health services, which have no cost and utilization control, and of HMO health services, which restrict choice of providers and have the usual panoply of management controls on utilization.

The growth of PPOs has been nothing short of phenomenal. PPO enrollees and their dependents numbered 1.3 million at the end of 1984, 5.8 million by mid-1985, 16.5 million by mid-1986 (Gabel and Ermann, 1985; de Lissovoy, Rice, Gabel, and Gelzer, 1987), and over double that number by mid-1988 (Rice and others, 1989). Whereas there were virtually no PPOs in the early 1980s, by mid-1988, 660 PPOs were in existence. Although there is debate about the future of PPOs and whether they contain health care costs and control physician and client behavior, their existence, ephemeral or permanent, underlines the depiction of the 1980s health care environment as a fecund spawning ground for new organizational forms.

Yet, in the midst of unprecedented organizational innovation, change, and experimentation, organizational weakness and failure have also become commonplace. With some exceptions, the subsector of rural hospitals has experienced levels of instability not seen since the Great Depression; many have closed entirely. Inner-city public hospitals, too, have had unusually difficult problems along with falling performance levels. Experiments in diversification and vertical integration have been abruptly terminated, with parent corporate organizations closing, selling, and converting satellite primary-care clinics and smaller hospitals. In the latter part of the 1980s, HMOs, despite previous strong growth, performed poorly financially, many recording substantial losses.

These successes and failures have occurred in a financial environment almost out of control: Total expenditures for health care were $248 billion in 1980 and approximately $647 billion in 1990, per capita expenditures increasing from $1,353 to $2,353 as measured in 1985 dollars. The average cost per hospital day, again in 1985 dollars, was a little over $300 in 1980, but over $700 in 1990. The percentage of the gross national product spent on health care was about 9.5 in 1980; it rose to about 11.5 in 1990. By 1984 health care was the third largest industry in the United States, after food and housing (data from Stoline and Weiner, 1988).

Underlying Forces

Large and increasing expenditures and other environmental turbulences have many causes, as the authors in this book emphasize. It is useful to review a number of these causes here, but readers are advised to consult other sources for detailed treatments (for example, Anderson, Lave, Russe, and Neuman, 1989; Stoline and Weiner, 1988). First, reimbursement for much hospital care has undergone dramatic change, largely as an attempt to stem expenditures, particularly in acute-care short-stay hospitals. Prospective reimbursement linked with a case-mix methodology (diagnosis-related groups in the case of Medicare) was but the first instance of limits placed by third-party insurers, including state Medicaid programs, on the total amount of money they will pay for hospital, and increasingly for medical, services.

The large infusion of complex technologies is a second force that has contributed to change in the health care environment. From implantable heart defibrillators and mobile lithotrypsy units (noninvasive treatment for kidney stones) to computerized tomography scanners, magnetic-resonance-imaging units, and a host of surgical advances, new techniques and devices have been introduced and adopted at an astounding rate. No sooner does a hospital or physician group acquire a new instrument than it must be replaced by a more effective one. Such advances whet the public's appetite for more of these technological miracles, and the demand increases as expectations rise. All these factors constitute a third force for change. Providers, wary of accusations of malpractice and poor quality of care, eagerly embrace the new technologies, and the ever-expanding spiral of introduction and adoption completes one more loop.

A fourth force is the agendas of state rate-setting commissions, which have constrained hospital discretion. These programs are designed to restrict the prices hospitals may charge; price limits and reimbursement ceilings are typical mechanisms.

A fifth force is the playing out of the unparalleled growth in hospitals from the late 1940s to the 1970s; redundant capacity led to competition for patients (Stevens, 1989). This oversupply of beds has been exacerbated by the effect of cost-control-minded reimbursement policies: dramatic declines in hospital admissions, fewer in-patient days, shorter lengths of stay, and lower occupancy rates, which fell from about 74 percent in 1983 to about 63 percent in 1985.

A sixth force that has altered the hospital environment is the emergence of a possibly less recalcitrant and more compliant physician work force. The abundance of physicians (from about 200 active physicians per 100,000 population in 1980 to about 230 per 100,000 in 1990) and the heightened costs of medical education are two causes of this change. Also contributing to the potentially more malleable work force is the presence of foreign medical graduates, comprising fully one-fifth of all physicians, many of whom are more willing to practice in settings traditionally eschewed by U.S.-educated physicians. A greater proportion of women are physicians than in the 1970s, but they continue to bear the brunt of household duties and thus often prefer regular, fixed working schedules that are made to order for administrators seeking full-time salaried medical personnel. And, finally, the respectability of the medical profession has diminished in the public's view as measured by many opinion surveys. Hence, there has been a decline in the ability of organized medicine to effect changes in medical manpower policy.

A seventh force is the aging of the U.S. population, which necessitates additional chronic-care services, long-term-care facilities, and durable medical equipment. But the squeeze on insurance systems, the abrupt repeal of Medicare catastrophic insurance, and the low profit margins of nursing homes make expansion in this sector problematical. An eighth force is the unprecedented risk and increasing costs of acquired immune deficiency syndrome, with the typical patient costing more than $100,000 to care for.

These and other forces have led to the kinds of environmental changes already described; these changes are often apparently contradictory: organizational downsizing coterminous with growth of new organizational forms, a surplus of physicians coupled with a shortage of nurses, cost-cutting efforts along with pressure for increasing insurance coverage, slackening of basic health-status indicators concurrent with near-miraculous capabilities to save life in the direst situations of disease and trauma.

From Health Care System to Healthcare Industry

To appreciate the profoundness of these changes, one needs only to examine a key difference in the labeling of health care in the 1980s compared with the labeling in previous decades: the penchant of writers to substitute the term *healthcare industry* for *health care system* or *medical care system*. The previous terms implied, in part, that all the disparate parts in the system had logical and rational interconnections and links. One had the sense that by careful study and analysis the nature of these interconnections and their causal influence on one another could be described. Careful study and analysis, in turn, could lead to rational intervention to change aspects of the health care system and could help predict the effects of such intervention. The tools of rational intervention were planning, problem identification, administrative control, and coordination. These notions fit well into an intellectual and political climate that fostered the belief that rational activity by government could solve a host of problems—a shortage of hospital beds, a shortage and maldistribution of physicians, limited access to services by the poor, and so forth. Finally, use of the term *medical* instead of *health* underscored the central role of the physician.

The current term, *healthcare industry,* is striking because it makes health care a single word. Although the form may not be correct, this word is a powerful symbol of the transition from system to industry. (The term *medical care* was, by contrast, never made into a single word.) Healthcare invites a crisp, avant-garde view of current reality, connoting efficiency and corporate expertise.

Substituting *industry* for *system* connotes much more. First, it reflects the explicit use of economic criteria in evaluating the performance of organizations and individuals who provide health services. Second, it signals an important shift in the thinking of many that health care organizations, physicians, nurses, and others are engaged essentially in the exchange of services in economic markets. They are thus subject to the forces of supply and demand as well as to distortions in market efficiency induced by governmental interference, monopoly (seller or producer) and monopsony (buyer or consumer) power, consumer ignorance, fetters to price sensitivity, and the like. Third, although the switch in terms does not deny irrational choice in health care activities, it elevates the importance of rationality among individual consumers and producers of health care. Fourth, it increases the salience of for-profit organizations. Large national and transnational health-delivery organizations, with securities traded on the major stock exchanges, move to center stage. Entrepreneurs take on important new roles as purveyors of medical technology; as brokers in complicated contractual arrangements among employers, insurers, beneficiaries, delivery organizations, and health professionals; and as consultants.

Fifth, *industry* suggests that intervention, if there be any at all, should remove barriers to the free movement of forces in mar-

ketplaces. Hence, antitrust activities have assumed a new importance in the health care industry.

Sixth, the industrial model emphasizes consumers rather than
patients, producers and providers rather than doctors and nurses.
Wants and desires replace needs; marketing replaces needs assessment
and epidemiology; market segment replaces subpopulation.

Seventh, the shift from system to industry may be as much
a change in locus of control as it is a shift from government fiat to
free markets. As Starr (1982, p. 449) argues, "The failure to rationalize medical services under public control meant that sooner or later
they would be rationalized under private control. Instead of public
regulation, there will be private regulation, and instead of public
planning, there will be corporate planning."

In addition to the fact that market actions produce conditions that require new strategies on the part of organizational managers and physicians, decision-making power appears to have
shifted from public to private entities. At the least, private involvement in health care, present since well before the twentieth century,
has taken additional forms that mimic private corporate structures.

Yet the diminishing role of government may be more appearance than reality. Arnould and DeBrock (1986, p. 284) note that "the
increased emphasis on government policies and private reimbursement mechanisms that place greater reliance on appropriate market
incentives by altering the behavior of providers is a recent phenomenon which has emerged almost simultaneously with increased state
regulation of hospital rates." Thus, active governmental intervention has been aimed at removing barriers historically leading to
market failure. Such intervention has taken the form of active support of HMOs, which collect fixed fees from members for a comprehensive set of medical and health services, and it has supported
other financing and organizational structures meant to provide economic incentives for efficient use of services. However, large employers and employer groups, major health insurers, and others in
the private sector have also attempted to promote similar goals. In
addition, some states have increased their regulatory activities
through rate-setting commissions at the same time that other states
have restricted and even abandoned their health-systems agencies
and certificate-of-need programs. Hence, as Arnould and DeBrock

note, it is difficult to separate the effects, if any, of deregulation and reregulation.

From Health Care Environments to
Organization Theory: Themes

From out of this confused and, some argue, uncontrolled environment comes grist for the mill of the analysts of health care organizations. The authors in this book have grappled with four major themes: the complexity of organizational environments, organizational innovation, strategic activity, and transaction-cost economics. I examine here each of these themes to underscore certain convergences and also to reveal differences and disagreements that are not always so clear.

Organizational Environments. Because this book was written in part to describe the impact of changes in the environment on health care organizations, it should not come as a surprise that all the chapters include depictions or assessments of the environment to a greater or lesser degree. It should also not be a surprise that different authors have different views on the importance of the environment in explaining organizational behavior. However, there is more convergence around two features of the environment than might be expected: the interactive nature of environmental components and the complex nature of organizational environments.

In regard to the first feature, the reader will discover that a duality exists in these chapters. On the one hand, there is an emphasis on objective, macrolevel forces that act deterministically on organizations. On the other hand, there is the view that voluntaristic managerial discretion plays a role in shaping environments. Hannan and Freeman (1989), in summarizing their organization ecology program, make perhaps the strongest statement yet in favor of the influence of deterministic, macrolevel forces on organizational change. None of the authors in this book makes such a radical statement, and most would not agree that organization theory is somehow compromised or necessarily made anthropomorphic because one considers the effect of individual actions, especially strategic actions, on organizations. The strongest statements in favor of strategy—Chapters Five, Six, Eight—would argue that managers can effect changes, intended and unintended, in environments, and would insist that theory incorporate nonrecursive (feedback or reciprocal-causation) links between the environment and managerial action.

The institutional perspectives of Richard Scott and Elaine Backman (Chapter Two) as well as of Jeffrey Alexander and Thomas D'Aunno (Chapter Three) seem to downplay voluntaristic behavior and question the importance of managerial discretion in strong technical and institutional environments. Yet, Alexander and D'Aunno's effort to explain change in the environments themselves may actually emphasize the nonrecursive relationship between organization and actor. If, as they argue, environments are influenced by changes in the relative strength of technical versus institutional demands and by shifts in the beliefs held by important groups in organizations, then theorists can see how the organizations themselves can alter their environments through, for example, political lobbying and the exertion of pressure to change regulatory agencies, including changes in their leadership.

Conscious attempts to change the environment do not mean, however, that intended outcomes of discretionary behavior result in actual outcomes; the point is simply that environments are not themselves completely uncontrolled, unfathomable forces. One could even argue that organizational ecology, for all its emphasis on organizational passivity, chance, and lottery, does not explain how and why the environments themselves change, a critical part of that theoretical approach (for if environments do not change, then organizations cannot be expected to change). The various views on strategic management suggest that at both the aggregate and the individual organizational levels, discretionary activities— technology acquisition, vertical integration, case management, to name several presented in this book—ultimately affect the environment itself. Hence, the time is past for simple models of one-way influence or causation between organization and environment; feedback loops and simultaneity, or mutual causation, should be considered.

An emphasis on the complexity of environments may not be as surprising as I suggested given the many published descriptions of the health care environment's multifarious characteristics. However, as an analytical device, organizational environments have generally been viewed in relatively simple ways. Some chapters in this book suggest that parsimony in this area may be premature. Two of those dealing with organizational innovation—Chapters Four and Seven—underscore the idea that the complexity of the environment is, in fact, the important conceptual piece in the puzzle of organizational innovation.

Other chapters reinforce this theme. Scott and Backman's thesis (Chapter Two) is that a theory of health care organization decoupled from the singular dominance of medical professionals has opened up serious consideration of other forces that shape organizations. This perspective, allied with some of Scott's work in sector theory (Scott and Meyer, 1983; Scott and Lammers, 1985), pushes us toward an examination not only of the complexity of organizational environments but also of the patterns of organization, particularly hierarchical relationships, among the relevant entities. Arnold Kaluzny, Joseph Morrissey, and Martha McKinney present in Chapter Four a parallel idea—that there are gains to be made by considering the rise of new organizational forms as the result of the interaction of organizations within administratively multitiered contexts. And when Stephen Shortell and Edward Zajac (Chapter Six) emphasize the importance of strategic alliances among health care organizations, they are also proposing that systems and networks are the key to a full understanding of organizational adaptation to environmental change. Finally, I argue in Chapter Eight that only through a decomposition of environment can the opposing theories of transaction-cost economics and strategic management be synthesized.

I as well as most of the other authors suggest specific research activities, but underlying all our perspectives is the message that more theoretical order needs to be brought to the study of organizational environments, and the work on the subject that began in the 1960s must continue.

Organizational Innovation. Three chapters make contributions to the discussion of organizational innovation, and three particular theoretical problems surface. First, how do new organizations emerge, without precedent and history, melding actors who have not traditionally been particularly cooperative (for example, community physicians and medical-center research physician-scientists)? Second, what can explain the concurrent appearance of new medical technology and organizational arrangements specifically designed to adopt the innovative technology? In short, what theoretical position can interpret simultaneous technological and organizational innovation? Third, what approach or approaches might one use to explain some of the innovative hospital/physician relationships that emerged in the 1980s and that have no strong historical antecedent?

To answer the first question, Kaluzny, Morrissey, and McKinney (Chapter Four) present an amalgamation of two theoretical views, an interaction model and a type of "value-added" approach to innovation in which a particular arrangement of forces or preconditions is hypothesized. The second question is tackled by Laura Renshaw, John Kimberly, and Sanford Schwartz (Chapter Seven) through a recasting of organizational-ecology theory and standard diffusion theory in which initiatives by managers, medical practitioners, and entrepreneurs count heavily. The third question, addressed by James Begun, Roice Luke, and Dennis Pointer (Chapter Five), is placed in the context of organizational structure and strategic purpose.

These three chapters aim at understanding how in one decade a welter of new organizational forms was able to arise. The approaches are interconnected because Chapter Four suggests the factors needed to permit the establishment of a new organizational arrangement that will coordinate activities by disparate actors, while Chapter Five suggests that the overarching strategic purpose of the actors can be a key to understanding innovative organizational forms. Chapter Seven directs attention to organizational adoption of innovation but adds the twist that organizations doing the adopting are themselves innovations introduced to allow the acquisition of technology.

No obvious synthesis of the authors' various solutions is possible, and none will be attempted here. However, the research agenda that each chapter proposes implicitly and explicitly offers some insight into areas where additional work is needed. Kaluzny,

Morrissey, and McKinney (Chapter Four) suggest that organizational innovation can be enhanced through interorganizational networks rather than through a process embedded within a single organization. Determining whether conventional approaches to innovation are obsolete or incomplete would be part of the challenge for researchers.

In their venturesome chapter, Renshaw, Kimberly, and Schwartz (Chapter Seven) press the case for further research into technology adoption because, given the unusual organizational arrangements and interactions in the spread of magnetic-resonance-imaging units, it is clear that conventional depictions of organizational innovation are not sufficiently explanatory. Thus, independently of Kaluzny, Morrissey, and McKinney, they also maintain that research on innovation should be conducted at an interorganizational level and with particular attention to the nature of the markets involved.

And, finally, Begun, Luke, and Pointer (Chapter Five) are explicit about the importance of taking organizational interdependence into account when devising explanations for the rise of new organizational forms. Their model is, in fact, a classification of types of organizational interdependence, and they believe that interorganizational networks are necessary conditions for innovation. Their research agenda stresses the need, first, for careful and refined identification and classification of organizational/professional relationships. Second, the nature of such interdependence needs investigation; is it reciprocal or sequential? Third, researchers need to determine how differences in strategic purpose and type of organizational "coupling" are measured.

These three approaches reveal a common concern with organizational interpenetration and interorganizational bases of innovation. All urge research in this relatively undeveloped area.

Strategic Activity. Clearly, strategic activity is encountered in each of the chapters just discussed. Mandates for Kaluzny, Morrissey, and McKinney's Community Clinical Oncology Program (Chapter Four) come from programmatic federal goals, which are buttressed by substantial funding. Strategic purpose of actors is central for Begun, Luke, and Pointer's typology (Chapter Five), which

breaks health care organizations into four distinct types. And investment, prestige, and clinician desire for the most modern diagnostic
and treatment processes are clearly strategic rationales for the acquisition and use of magnetic resonance imaging, as Renshaw, Kimberly, and Schwartz (Chapter Seven) demonstrate.

But Chapter Six makes the strongest case for bringing strategic action into organization theory. Shortell and Zajac assert that
if sense is to be made out of the adaptation of health care organizations to the turbulent 1980s environment, it will be made
through a study of strategy. They "demystify" discussions of the
environment by proposing that environments are not monolithic
forces that cause either organizational conformity or demise but are
collections of organizations in a network relationship that contribute to a rich and complicated set of organizational outcomes.
Organizations may engage in strategic activity to alter these relationships and may thereby add to the overall turbulence and complexity of the environment. Thus, we see another conclusion in
favor of nonrecursive systems.

Shortell and Zajac propose an explicit research agenda that
stems from their theoretical synthesis of the literature on strategic
management. In a series of hypotheses, they suggest combining all
the component parts—environments, organizations, managers,
markets, and organizational performance—into a forward-looking
research agenda that urges bringing people back into organization
theory.

In almost all the other chapters also, there is a rethinking of
the place of discretion in organization theory. Begun, Luke, and
Pointer, (Chapter Five) place strategy on an equal footing with
structure in their classification scheme of organizational forms. In
Chapter Eight I counterpose strategy and transaction-cost economics to explain vertical integration. Such rethinking is probably a
function of the various authors' efforts to comprehend the immense
variation in organizational forms and performance in health care
during the 1980s. No environmentally deterministic model seems
sensitive enough by itself to explain this variation or to appreciate
the detail and variety that have emerged. Hence, all seek and urge
research that will continue to address this question, and some argue
that strategy may be the key to unraveling the mystery. At the very

least, the question of macrolevel forces versus the strategic will of people in shaping organizational forms and performance has been raised.

Transaction-Cost Economics. In the mid-1970s organization theorists read Williamson's (1975) thesis that transaction-cost economics could explain why organizations exist, not to mention why they integrate vertically. Not surprisingly, organization theorists have been reluctant for several reasons either to embrace the market-failures paradigm or to distinguish those elements that might fruitfully be integrated into existing or new organization theory. First, disputes exist about the relative influence of efficiency and power in explaining organizational behavior. Second, many organization theorists, especially those grounded in case studies and direct field experience, do not believe that organizations offer "frictionless" and efficient ways to produce goods and services. Third, the testy issue of how to measure transaction costs remains.

Despite these problems, Chapters Eight and Nine both try to integrate the transaction-cost perspective and organization theory. My research agenda (Chapter Eight) revolves around explicit hypotheses related to the relative influence of transaction costs, strategic purpose, and other factors in explaining vertical integration; the extent to which decision processes in vertical integration are motivated by transaction-cost reduction, holding production costs constant; and, more broadly, the effect of differentiated environmental and market circumstances on the relationship between transaction costs and strategic actions.

Robert Hurley and Mary Fennell (Chapter Nine) offer the tantalizing hypothesis that transaction costs may be lowered in so-called managed health care schemes because the integration of health care financing and delivery reduces costs that more traditional financing and delivery schemes have failed to lower. Although their case studies tend to support the notion, they offer a larger research agenda that encourages more formal examination of issues such as whether the putative cost savings of integrated transactions offset other costs that critics might ascribe to managed-care schemes. These other costs include reduction in client freedom of choice, less discretion for providers in making decisions about care, lower levels of access to both providers and delivery organizations by clients, and the imposition of penalties and exclusions of care for clients who fail to abide by the rules. Hurley and Fennell imply that such costs do not necessarily result when transaction-costs are lowered. The issue is a major empirical one with virtually no systematic research yet under way. The salience of the issue is high because both public and private insurers as well as other parties involved in the financing of health care (employers, unions, state and local governments) find the cost-savings promises of managed care interesting and attractive alternatives to traditional forms of financing (indemnity insurance) and delivering (fee-for-service) health care.

In both these chapters, the underlying empirical problem is how to measure transaction costs and to distinguish them from production costs. In Chapter Eight I assert that we are still far from close to agreement on this question, although internal transfer pricing is a possible avenue for study. Nevertheless, analysts will insist that we observe these costs directly and not infer that they exist, and hence we still have much to do in the measurement realm before transaction-cost analysis becomes an acceptable technique in organization theory.

Goals of This Book

Organization theory outside health care is experiencing a similar profusion of new views. It is difficult to find any of society's organizational sectors that have not been transformed recently by change; the varied perspectives of Burrell and Morgan (1979), Perrow (1986), Scott (1981, 1987), and Grandori (1987), among others, provide us with convenient summaries of the state of the field. Yet, despite different theoretical orientations, all would probably agree with Scott (1987, p. xv): "The field of organizations has undergone enormous change in the past few decades. It is currently, I believe, the most lively and vigorous area of study within sociology, and perhaps within all of the social sciences. This is a source of both excitement and confusion. Much is happening in the field, and developments are occurring faster than our ability to assimilate them into coherent patterns."

I believe this is also an apt description of the ferment in health care organization theory. It is, in addition, a reason not to overstate similarities and convergences among the various authors and their chapters. It is premature to place a template on what is still exploratory. In some areas a heavier editorial hand might also obscure some undeveloped interconnections. For example, could transaction-cost analysis be applied to Kaluzny, Morrissey, and McKinney's Community Clinical Oncology Program (Chapter Four)? In other words, are efficiencies gained by introduction of this novel organizational form because the environment is so uncertain and unstable? Or is efficiency an irrelevant consideration? Is effectiveness the overriding concern? This book is filled with such speculative possibilities.

In one's attempt to make sense of the diversity and complexity of the ideas expressed in this book, one could easily overemphasize simplistic themes and lose the heuristic value and creative tension that exist when there is disagreement. As is underscored by Poole and Van de Ven (1989), these disagreements—paradoxes—raise new questions and foreshadow new research agendas. Our hope is that by examining old organizations through new lenses and new organizations through old lenses in this book, we will offer deepened and helpful insights into organization theory and contribute to the field's growth and maturation.

References

Anderson, G. F., Lave, J. R., Russe, C. M., and Neuman, P. *Providing Hospital Services: The Changing Financial Environment.* Baltimore: Johns Hopkins University Press, 1989.

Arnould, R. J., and DeBrock, L. M. "Competition and Market Failure in the Hospital Industry: A Review of the Evidence." *Medical Care Review*, 1986, *43* (2), 243–292.

Burrell, G., and Morgan, G. *Sociological Paradigms and Organizational Analysis.* London: Heinemann, 1979.

Croog, S. H., and Ver Steeg, D. F. "The Hospital as a Social System." In H. E. Freeman, S. Levine, and L. G. Reeder (eds.), *Handbook of Medical Sociology* (2nd ed.). Englewood Cliffs, N.J.: Prentice-Hall, 1972.

de Lissovoy, G., Rice, T., Ermann, D., and Gabel, J. "Preferred Provider Organizations: Today's Models and Tomorrow's Prospects." *Inquiry*, 1986, *23*, 7–15.

de Lissovoy, G., Rice, T., Gabel, J., and Gelzer, H. "Preferred Provider Organizations: One Year Later." *Inquiry*, 1987, *24*, 127–136.

Duff, R. S., and Hollingshead, A. B. *Sickness and Society*. New York: Harper & Row, 1968.

Feldman, R., Kralewski, J., and Dowd, B. "Health Maintenance Oganizations: The Beginning or the End?" *Health Services Research*, 1989, *24* (2), 191–211.

Fox, R. C. *Experiment Perilous: Physicians and Patients Facing the Unknown*. New York: Free Press, 1959.

Freidson, E. *Doctoring Together: A Study of Professional Social Control*. New York: Elsevier Science, 1975.

Gabel, J., and Ermann, D. "Preferred Provider Organizations: Performance, Problems and Promise." *Health Affairs*, 1985, *4*, 24–40.

Georgopoulos, B. S. *Hospital Organization Research: Review and Source Book*. Philadelphia: Saunders, 1975.

Goffman, E. *Asylums: Essays on the Social Situation of Mental Patients and Other Inmates*. New York: Doubleday, 1961.

Grandori, A. *Perspectives on Organization Theory*. Cambridge, Mass.: Ballinger, 1987.

Hannan, M. T., and Freeman, J. *Organizational Ecology*. Cambridge, Mass.: Harvard University Press, 1989.

Kimberly, J. R. "The Design of Health Care Organizations." In B. Fetter, J. D. Thompson, and J. R. Kimberly (eds.), *Cases in Health Management and Policy*. Homewood, Ill.: Irwin, 1985.

Levine, S., and White, P. E. "Exchange as a Conceptual Framework for the Study of Interorganizational Relationships." *Administrative Science Quarterly*, 1961, *5*, 583–597.

Levine, S., White, P. E., and Paul, B. D. "The Community of Health Organizations." In H. E. Freeman, S. Levine, and L. G. Reeder (eds.), *Handbook of Medical Sociology* (2nd ed.). Englewood Cliffs, N.J.: Prentice-Hall, 1972.

Levine, S., White, P. E., and Paul, B. D. "Community Interorganizational Problems in Providing Medical Care and Social Services." *American Journal of Public Health*, 1963, *53*, 1183–1219.

Milner, M., Jr. *Unequal Care: A Case Study of Interorganizational Relations in Health Care.* New York: Columbia University Press, 1980.

Perrow, C. "The Analysis of Goals in Complex Organizations." *American Sociological Review*, 1961, *26*, 854–866.

Perrow, C. *Complex Organizations: A Critical Essay.* (3rd ed.). New York: Random House, 1986.

Poole, M. S., and Van de Ven, A. H. "Using Paradox to Build Management and Organization Theory." *Academy of Management Review*, 1989, *14* (4), 562–578.

Rice, T., and others. *PPOs: Bigger, Not Better.* Research Bulletin R989. Washington, D.C.: Health Insurance Association of America, 1989.

Scott, W. R. "Developments in Organization Theory, 1960–1980." *American Behavioral Scientist*, 1981, *24* (3), 407–422.

Scott, W. R. *Organizations: Rational, Natural, and Open Systems.* (2nd ed.). Englewood Cliffs, N.J.: Prentice-Hall, 1987.

Scott, W. R., and Lammers, J. C. "Trends in Occupations and Organizations in the Medical Care and Mental Health Sectors." *Medical Care Review*, 1985, *42*, 37–76.

Scott, W. R., and Meyer, J. W. "The Organization of Societal Sectors." In J. W. Meyer and W. R. Scott (eds.), *Organizational Environments: Ritual and Rationality.* Beverly Hills, Calif.: Sage, 1983.

Shortell, S. M., and Kaluzny, A. D. *Health Care Management: A Text in Organization Theory and Behavior.* (2nd ed.). New York: Wiley, 1988.

Starr, P. *The Social Transformation of American Medicine.* New York: Basic Books, 1982.

Stevens, R. *In Sickness and in Wealth: American Hospitals in the Twentieth Century.* New York: Basic Books, 1989.

Stoline, A., and Weiner, J. P. *The New Medical Marketplace: A Physician's Guide to the Health Care Revolution.* Baltimore: Johns Hopkins University Press, 1988.

Williamson, O. E. *Markets and Hierarchies: Analysis and Antitrust Implications.* New York: Free Press, 1975.

2

Institutional Theory
and the Medical Care Sector

W. Richard Scott
Elaine V. Backman

In the first part of this chapter, we look back at early theory and research by sociologists who examined the nature of work and the organization of work within the medical care sector (although the notion of sector was developed late in the period we cover). We review past work in order to understand better changes in organizational arrangements as well as changes in our conceptions of these arrangements. In particular, we examine the roots and nutrients of the institutional perspective. As nicely dramatized by the movie *Back to the Future,* our view of the past is altered when we examine it having knowledge of the future—that is, our present.

In the second part of the chapter, we shift from reviewing the past to forecasting the future. We suggest that the current discourse on ethics in medical care provides a fertile ground for investigation by researchers working within the institutional perspective.

Note: Earlier versions of this chapter were presented at the annual meeting of the American Sociological Association, San Francisco, Aug. 1989, and at a conference on "Advancing Institutional Theory," University of Michigan, Ann Arbor, June 1989.

We acknowledge the collaboration and comments of John W. Meyer and the helpful comments of Walter W. Powell.

This chapter was completed while Scott was a Fellow at the Center for Advanced Study in the Behavioral Sciences. He is grateful for the financial support provided by the John D. and Catherine T. MacArthur Foundation.

LOOKING BACKWARD: SOURCES OF THE
INSTITUTIONAL PERSPECTIVE

Focus on the Professions

Sociologists noticed quite early that the medical care sector was not organized in the same manner as most other arenas involving complex work. In attempting to account for the differences in organizational forms, early students emphasized the importance of professional occupations within the sector. Parsons (1939) and Hughes (1958) were only the best known of a large number of analysts who stressed the central role played by professionals in defining the nature of the work to be performed and the proper division of labor, in setting standards for evaluating successful performance, and in determining appropriate control and support structures. Freidson (1970a, p. 77) makes explicit the primary assumption guiding this work when he asserts: "The most important single element in the social structure of medical care is the medical profession itself."

Professions Versus Other Occupations. Much attention has been lavished on professional occupations, and the assumptions and foci guiding investigations have changed over time. In the first stage of this work, the central comparisons were among occupations: How did professions differ from other types of occupations? During this period, sociological work on the professions proceeded at two levels of analysis: the structural and the social-psychological, with social-psychological analysis focusing on the socialization of individuals into professional roles. Present purposes are served, however, by restricting attention to structural approaches. At this level, we can note three trends: the shift from a generic to a more differentiated model of the professions; a shift from ahistoric to more historically sensitive models; and a shift from functionalist to power or conflict assumptions.

From Carr-Saunders and Wilson's (1933) early discussion to Freidson's latest reexamination (1986), observers have been preoccupied with identifying characteristics that distinguish professions from other occupations, with analysts giving varying emphasis to a larger or smaller set of such characteristics. Among the character-istics included on most lists were: (1) practice is based on a body of general, systematic knowledge; (2) practitioners assert the need for autonomy in decision making—in particular, protection from non-professional controls; and (3) norms are espoused that support al-truism or a service orientation. (See, for example, Greenwood, 1957; Goode, 1957; Hughes, 1958; Parsons, 1939.) This early work as-sumed that a single generic model covered all professional occupa-tions; disagreements centered on the number, definition, and relative importance of the distinguishing features.

As Abbott (1988) emphasizes, early observers of the medical scene were particularly prone to embrace the assumption of a ge-neric model: Their attention was focused on one profession—med-icine—and one context—the United States.

Closely related to the search for a generic model of the pro-fessions was the assumption of ahistoricity. Just as the early analysts attempted to identify a single ideal model, ignoring differences within and among the professions, so did they also deemphasize changes over time. When they did recognize historical change, more often than not they believed that such change was a one-way, lock-step process, and they regarded different professions as being at different "stages of development" (see, for example, Caplow, 1954).

Only since the 1960s have analysts begun to take seriously differences within and among professional occupations and to examine changes over time in their distinctive features. Some exam-ined differences among the subgroups or specialties within profes-sions (for example, Smith, 1958; Bucher and Strauss, 1961); others called attention to changes over time in professionalization pro-cesses (for example, Millerson, 1964; Wilensky, 1964); and still oth-ers began systematically to examine relations among varying professional occupations and to explore differences in the charac-teristics of professions depending on when, where, and how they developed (for example, Jackson, 1970; Larson, 1977). We discuss these developments more fully later in the chapter.

At about the same time that analysts were embracing differ-entiated and historically sensitive models, a shift occurred in the kinds of assumptions made concerning the causal processes at work in the construction and maintenance of professional occupations. Early explanations of the distinctive features of the professions assumed a functionalist stance: Professional structures arose as solutions to problems; general, systematic knowledge was required to deal with unusually complex problems; collegial controls were necessary because nonprofessionals could not evaluate the quality of the work being performed; altruistic norms were necessary to ensure that practitioners would not exploit dependent recipients of services. Such arguments stressed the value of professional forms to client interests or to the wider community. (See, for example, Parsons, 1939; Goode, 1957.)

By contrast, the newer work emphasized the benefits associated with professional forms to the professionals themselves and attempted to examine the mechanisms by which occupational groups acquired sufficient power to enforce their monopoly position and escape external controls. Among the strategies and tactics stressed as central to the acquisition of power were the devising of ideological arguments that emphasize the importance of the services provided and the complexity and uncertainty of the work performed and the acquiring of state support for exclusive jurisdiction over specified types of work or occupational titles (Freidson, 1970b, 1986; Johnson, 1972; Larson, 1977; Abbott, 1988). We will return to these arguments about the role of power after we review a parallel line of developing theory and research.

Professions Versus Bureaucracy. A second line of investigation developed alongside that examining differences between professions and other occupations. In this approach, the professions were compared with administrative forms or, as more commonly phrased, with bureaucracy. As with the first type of inquiry, this work also proceeded at both the structural and the social-psychological levels. Here, however, both levels have relevance to the present discussion. Early work was conducted at the social-psychological level.

During the late 1950s, several investigators noted that although an increasing number of professionals were no longer operating as independent practitioners but as employees of organizations, they often did not behave as conventional employees.

They exhibited considerable independence: They were more likely to be guided by the norms and standards of collegial groups beyond organizational boundaries; they were more oriented to the development and exercise of their distinctive skills than to advancement in the organizational hierarchy; they were likely to consider career moves between organizations rather than developing commitments to a specific organization. (See, for example, Bennis, Berkowitz, Affinito, and Malone, 1958; Gouldner, 1957–1958; Wilensky, 1956.) These studies were significant in that they were among the first to demonstrate that work-relevant expectations and behavior of organizational employees could be shaped by groups independent of and external to the control structures of the immediate, employing organization.

Studies of varying role orientations exhibited by professionals quickly led to the insight that what was at issue was not simply differences in role definition among individual employees but contrasting social structures. For example, Kornhauser (1962, p. 8) pointed out that in examining the behavior of professionals in bureaucracies, we are probing "the relation between two institutions, not merely between organizations and individuals." (See also Blau and Scott, 1962, p. 60.) Investigators began to recognize that the two systems represented alternative models for rationalizing complex work (Scott, 1966; Hall, 1968; Freidson, 1973).

Researchers noted variations in mechanisms for achieving rationality. Professional models emphasize the development of general theoretical frameworks from which principles are derived to guide the selection of activities to be carried out by broadly trained, flexible performers having command of a wide repertoire of performance programs. The autonomy of these individual performers and their commensurate responsibility for choices made are stressed. Bureaucratic approaches also posit the desirability of a general framework to guide the conduct of activities but emphasize the advantages of both horizontal and vertical differentiation: A horizontal division of labor provides the benefits associated with task specialization; the vertical division of control permits a few higher-level participants to plan, oversee, and coordinate the work of a larger set of lower-level participants. In the bureaucratic model, decision making and control activities are centralized and the autonomy of lower-level participants is restricted. Despite differences in the mechanisms employed, both models rest on a common conception of the desirability of operating within a rationalized field of activity.

Pioneer studies of professional/bureaucratic relations tended to assume that just as there was one model of the profession, there was one ideal-typical model of bureaucracy. Gradually, empirical research demonstrated a wide variety of organizational structures and a similarly wide range of professional adaptations (Kornhauser, 1962; Vollmer and Mills, 1966). Bureaucratic forces dominate in some situations. Labeled "heteronomous" professional organizations, these bureaucracies circumscribed the discretion exercised by professional employees and use routine hierarchical supervision. Public social welfare agencies, elementary and secondary schools, and mental health organizations are likely to have these characteristics. Professional influences dominate in other situations. Labeled "autonomous" professional organizations, they have professional employees who organized themselves into a corporate body to define and defend an enlarged sphere of autonomy from administrative encroachment. Universities, hospitals, and law firms generally exhibit these features (Scott, 1965; 1982b; Hall, 1968; Etzioni, 1969; Larson, 1977). This line of argument and research established the existence of substantial variations in the organizational forms within which professionals worked and suggested that the more autonomous forms were associated with the more fully developed and powerful professions.

Finally, early analysts emphasized the conflicts and incompatibilities between professional and bureaucratic systems, whereas later work increasingly recognized the amount of overlap in their underlying assumptions and the various mechanisms fostering accommodation within functioning organizations.

To see the professional and bureaucratic forms as alternative means of rationalizing action, to observe that under many conditions professional actors are able to function within—indeed, are indispensable to—organizational systems, and to recognize that these actors are often more oriented to and governed by external professional structures than by the immediate administrative systems—these were important steps on the road to a broad perspective.

Incorporating Professions in Organizational Environments

A number of additional developments were required before analysts of the medical care sector could, to a degree, defocalize the medical profession and begin to acknowledge the effects of other actors and factors and thus to develop a broad analytic framework. These developments included shifting the focus from too exclusive a concern with structures at the level of the individual organization or the single professional occupation, placing individual professions in the broad context of competing occupations and supportive structures, and retrieving some of the insights of the functionalist perspective.

Shifting Attention to Wider Structures. Both organizational and professional forms operate at many levels. At the most general level, as already noted, each may be viewed as constituting alternative models—different cultural conceptions—of how to rationalize an arena of action. Each provides a theory or principles for establishing a division of labor, control arrangements, and systems of accountability. Concrete organizations and concrete professional occupations draw on and are sustained by these cultural patterns.

Although the models differ, they are not incompatible. Thus we observe in modern societies that the continuing evolution of bureaucracies has not supplanted or weakened the development of professions. Both have flourished, and they appear to be nurtured and supported by the same forces.

We have observed that the two forms often coexist in the same organization. At a more general level and in a rather metaphorical sense, we suggest that the two bases of organizing may be conceived as a macromatrix structure, in which occupations are differentiated while organizations function as project teams—units that select and deploy representatives of several occupations in varying arrangements to perform particular, interdependent tasks. (For a related discussion, see Clark, 1983.) And, as with the conventional matrix forms found in specific organizations, we observe the simultaneous existence of two rationales for control and two lines of authority impinging on a given actor.

Also, as concrete social structures, organizations and professional occupations are likely to have a number of levels. Groups of professional practitioners frequently organize themselves into a corporate body (for example, as a medical staff in a hospital or a faculty senate in a university) to make decisions and exercise collective control in particular organizational settings. Many such occupations develop structures to enable them to function at regional or state levels, the state being a highly salient environment in the United States for occupations seeking licensure. And these same occupations often have corporate bodies, such as associations or unions, organized to operate at the national or societal level. Similarly, an increasing number of organizations belong to large corporations that operate at multiple levels and sites, so that the individual establishment is embedded in an organization, and is influenced by events, remote from its immediate environment. Occupational and organizational forms at the several levels interact with and interpenetrate each other.

The adoption during the late 1960s and 1970s of the open-systems paradigm in organization theory has emphasized the sensitivity of intraorganizational structures and activities to extraorganizational forces and events. More recent theoretical and empirical work has stressed the variety of salient external factors and the multiple levels at which they operate. (For a review, see Scott, 1987b, pp. 119–142.) At the heart of an open-systems perspective, however, is the recognition that environmental factors are not to be regarded only or primarily as forces external to the organization. Rather, environmental inputs become ingredients of organizations: They penetrate them, thereby providing elements that constitute them. Thus elements of occupational groups can enter into and become components of organizations. We discuss later reasons why the incorporation of professionals into organizations occurs.

Contextualizing Professions. As noted, sociologists in the 1960s initiated a series of comparative and historically grounded studies. Led primarily by a new generation of researchers who rejected functionalism and sought to develop power explanations for professional prerogatives, sociologists began to study the ways in which numerous specific occupations acquired (or failed to acquire) their distinctive power and privileges or to examine variations in the experience of the same types of occupations operating in different societal contexts. (See, for example, Etzioni, 1969; Freidson, 1970b; Jackson, 1970; Stevens, 1971; Johnson, 1972; Rueschmeyer, 1973; Berlant, 1975.)

From these efforts, it gradually became apparent that an important aspect of the social context for any occupation is the number and nature of other occupations working in the same arena, related occupations with which it competes and coexists (Abbott, 1988). In some instances this competition is resolved in the sense that a relatively stable, sometimes elaborate, stratified hierarchy of dominant and ancillary occupations is created, with a relatively well-defined division of labor among them. This is by and large the situation in the medical care sector in the United States (Freidson, 1970a), although much jostling remains among the many segments and specialties within the medical profession (Bucher and Strauss, 1961; Stevens, 1971). In other situations no stable resolution develops, and competition—sometimes outright conflict—persists. The continuing battle among psychiatrists, psychologists, and social workers over domain definition and the appropriate division of tasks in the mental health arena is an example of such an unresolved controversy (Rushing, 1964; Foley and Sharfstein, 1983). A more recent instance of a jurisdictional dispute among professional groups is that between mental health practitioners and advocates of the Alcoholics Anonymous model for treatment of drug abuse (D'Aunno and Sutton, 1989).

More important, although previous students of the professions had noted that state power backed professional claims, little systematic attention was accorded to the role of the state in the professionalization process. Work has begun to correct this oversight. It is now recognized that nation-states differ greatly—both across societies and over time—in their willingness and capacity to support varying professions. Hence, when and where a profession develops significantly affect its position and prerogatives independently of knowledge base or technical prowess. Analysts such as Larson (1977), Fielding and Portwood (1980), Child and Fulk (1982), and Abbott (1988) have focused on profession/state connections, have illustrated the diversity of these ties, and have begun to create theories about these relationships.

Retrieving Insights from the Functionalist Perspective. The concerns first addressed by functionalist theorists were in retreat during the 1980s, drummed out by the competing assertions and interpretations of power theorists. It is important to distinguish, however, between the logic and the substance of arguments. Functionalist theorists were incorrect in attempting to account for the distinctive features of professions by pointing to their functions or consequences, but they were not wrong in calling attention to these distinguishing features. For example, most functionalist theories emphasized the importance of the values espoused by professionals: an interest in service to others. Although power theorists pointed out that professionals were not disinterested but were motivated by self-interest, the two motives are not necessarily in conflict. Indeed, Bledstein (1976) points out that the coexistence of self- and other interests constitutes one of the distinctive attributes of the "culture of professionalism." The combination of self-interest and service to others, of social advancement through social service, provides much of the appeal and the dynamism of the professions.

Functionalist theorists were also the first to call attention to the prominence of normative and cognitive elements in the construction and maintenance of professional communities. Many of their early insights have been dismissed or overshadowed by power models, but the institutionalist perspective has revived interest in these symbolic aspects of social structure. More so than many types of social systems, the professions rule by controlling belief systems. Their primary weapons are ideas. They exercise control by defining reality—by devising ontological frameworks, proposing distinctions, creating typifications, and fabricating principles or guidelines for action (Meyer, Boli, and Thomas, 1987).

Institutionalists side with the functionalists in recognizing the significance of symbolic features of professional systems; but they do not find it necessary to dismiss the insights of power theorists. Knowledge systems, like all belief systems, must be constructed and maintained, defended and extended. They have their advocates and their detractors, their creators and their critics. Their ascendancy benefits some and disadvantages or dispossesses other groups with conflicting claims. Analysts such as Ben-David (1963–1964), Bledstein (1976), Collins (1979), and Freidson (1986) are correct in emphasizing that the welfare and prospects of a profession are closely tied to its ability to develop effective links with centers of higher education—the principal organs in modern society of knowledge creation and transmission.

In short, it is as important to apply both a power and a functionalist perspective to the creation, maintenance, and dismantling of the symbolic systems on which professions rely as it is to apply them to the securing of state endorsements or market advantages. What Larson (1977) and DiMaggio (1982) refer to as the "professional project"—the task of putting into place the necessary infrastructure, connections among practitioners, and links with relevant constituencies and superstructures required to support and sustain a common enterprise—is a complex, prolonged, and indeed, never-ending pursuit.

More is involved than simply providing a valued service (the functionalist version) or creating a monopoly (the power version). Success depends on many factors, not the least of which is the cultivation of a knowledge base and theory of practice that instills confidence in providers and secures legitimacy among consumers. The institutionalization of such a base is a political process as well as an intellectual one.

Elaborating the Concept of Organizational Environments

The institutional perspective has sought to build on the insights of both functionalist and power theorists. Several trends that merit attention and require development are under way. We comment on four of these: an increasing awareness of the complexity of state/profession connections; a perception of environmental elements as independent as well as dependent variables; an expansion of the concept of power; and an examination of the connections between institutional and technical aspects of environments.

Expanding Models of State/Profession Relations. As we have described, students focusing on the historical development of the professions quickly encountered the state. We now need to examine the many facets of governments, the multiple mechanisms used by them to relate to professions, and the varying relations thus created.

Governments are often treated by analysts as if they were monolithic entities. In fact, most are more realistically viewed as highly differentiated, multifaceted, often loosely coupled congeries of organizations. Complex functions such as health and education are often spread across multiple semiautonomous agencies, which in some cases operate in complete ignorance of one another. Although in modern states welfare functions are increasingly centralized at the national level, high levels of differentiation and fragmentation exist there also (Meyer and Scott, 1983).

The backing of the state is necessary to secure a monopoly market position for an occupational group; such support involves giving exclusive access to an area of practice, jurisdiction over a class of activities, or, sometimes, only the right to the use of a designated occupational title. But the state can act in many other ways. It can subsidize research and training activities or stimulate the creation of particular types of provider arrangements (for example, health maintenance organizations). It can restrict employment in specified positions to those with particular professional credentials. And, of great importance now, it can insist that only those with appropriate professional certification be paid with state tax dollars for services provided.

In addition, the more powerful professions in modern society—such as medicine in the United States—are invited to share in the exercise of legitimate state power, and this role too can take a variety of forms: for example, proposing standards, drafting legislation, or being incorporated into implementation or review groups established to administer or oversee publicly mandated and funded programs (Alford, 1975; Starr, 1982). Most sociological observers today, particularly those embracing a power or conflict perspective, are highly suspicious and critical of such arrangements. They are clearly subject to abuse, but important benefits are associated with self-regulation; it needs to be contrasted not with an ideal model but with some feasible alternative control structure. Streeck and Schmitter (1985, p. 22) point out that, compared with conventional external regulatory bodies, professional control bodies enjoy distinct advantages because they "are closer to the target group (their members) than state bureaucracies, and they have more intimate knowledge of its situations and concerns. It is likely that this enables them to apply rules less formalistically and to take the specific conditions of individual cases into account—which in turn, tends to increase the acceptance of regulation by those affected by it."

The large number of public regulatory structures in the medical care sector that routinely include representatives of professional groups in their policy and implementation activities may be an indicator not only of the power of the professional groups but also of the astuteness of the regulatory agencies in recognizing the advantages of tapping into the competence and legitimacy of professional groups. The general point, however, is that state powers and privileges are likely to be widely distributed across the bureaucracy, may take many forms, and vary in their effects on professional position and practice.

Also, states are able to exercise power quite directly over a range of activities, not simply by supporting or curtailing the actions of particular professional groups. The single most important change in the medical care sector is the rapidly growing influence of governmental actors—in particular, federal agencies. From the Hill-Burton program in the mid-1940s through the passage of the Medicare and Medicaid programs in the mid-1960s to the current prospective-payment reimbursement scheme, the state has become a major player. State power has been employed to influence both the supply of medical services and the demand for them. Supply-side efforts include the Hill-Burton program to increase the number and change the distribution of hospital beds and recent attempts to increase the supply of physicians, in part to stimulate competitive forces. On the demand side, the U.S. government has become the largest single purchaser of medical care services. Although the state lacks the power to determine directly what services are to be provided, it can effectively shape the distribution of services by specifying the types and amounts of services for which it will pay.

Most analyses have emphasized the ways in which state power can be appropriated for professional projects, but states can also use their powers to curtail or undermine these interests. States can withhold legitimation from as well as award it to aspiring occupational groups: The complete history of the evolution of the medical care sector must include accounts of those occupations that failed to achieve state support as well as those that succeeded. The success of the medical physician in the United States is related to the failure of the Thomsonians, the Eclectics, the hydropaths, and the homeopaths (Abbott, 1988; Starr, 1982). States can also withdraw their support of groups previously anointed. Simon's (1983) account of the deprofessionalization of social workers in public agencies provides an illustration.

Even though nation-states may share with the professions a generalized interest in the rationalization of spheres of action, as DiMaggio and Powell (1983) have observed, they do not always agree on the preferred forms for achieving rational action. Persons wielding public power tend to favor centralized administrative forms, whereas professionals prefer decentralized structures that accord discretion to practitioners (Scott, 1987a). And, currently, many economically advanced nation-states are seeking increased efficiency and pressing for reforms by stimulating the private sector and by encouraging market forces. Such reform attempts often undermine professional prerogatives (Gray, 1986).

Environments as Independent Variables. Much effort has been expended and more is required to clarify the ways in which states, professions, and other collective actors interact to create distinctive institutional arrangements. But just as it is important to understand the causes of these arrangements and the forces that variously shape them, it is equally important that attention be given to their consequences. We need to examine institutions as both dependent and independent variables. The concept of institutional environment emphasizes the independent variables.

All the processes just described have important consequences for the structuring of the field of organizations—for the nature and number of various types of organizations that develop and for their interrelationships. For example, dissension and conflict over the professional division of labor or over appropriate treatment regimens will be reflected in interorganizational disputes over domain and the appropriate treatment of clients (Hall, 1986; D'Aunno and Sutton, 1989).

States also affect organizational fields. The ways in which the state exercises its power may be as significant as how much power it uses. As Meyer and Scott (Meyer, 1983; Scott and Meyer, 1983) note, in sectors dominated by professional providers, the U.S. government has exercised its influence primarily through funding controls rather than through direct efforts to command or proscribe specific actions; and it has carried out its activities by creating a large collection of loosely related and largely uncoordinated agencies and programs. These agencies have effects on the organizational field to which they relate. Control exercised by funding and reimbursement agencies expands the paraphernalia associated with accounting. The fragmentation of control agents gives rise to administrative buffers. Such buffers sometimes take the form of intermediate layers of administration—units mediating between funding and provider systems. And they sometimes exist as an elaborated administrative staff in each client organization, erected to deal with the multiple sources of resources (Bankston, 1982; Stackhouse, 1982; Meyer, Scott, and Strang, 1987).

Also, although the increase of corporations within the medical care sector surely has multiple causes, one salient cause probably is the increased complexity of the environment to which these organizations must relate. Corporate multihospital structures can more readily map and more effectively cope with complex fiscal and regulatory environments than can independent, freestanding hospitals (Alexander and Scott, 1984; Alexander and Amburgey, 1987).

Observers have also posited another, longer-term effect of public funding on the organization of the medical care sector. It has been argued that not only the vastly increased scale of funding but also the increased stability of funding has encouraged the reentry and rapid growth of all types of private, for-profit providers. (See, for example, Starr, 1982; Gray, 1986.) These developments have also been encouraged by the wave of deregulation activities and the encouragement of privatization efforts.

Thus significant changes have occurred in relations among the professions and between professions and states. These developments need to be analyzed and explained; their consequences for organizations and for the structure of organizational fields also merit our attention. Fortunately, during the 1980s both types of investigations were pursued.

Enlarging the Concept of Power. Among the most important contributions of recent institutional views is that they introduce new conceptions and arguments to help account for the behavior and structure of actors—both individual and corporate—in the health care sector. Many of these arguments, in a sense, hearken back to and rediscover some of the special features of professions that were dismissed or overshadowed when the power models displaced the functionalist conceptions.

The institutional persuasion gives renewed attention to the symbolic aspects of environments—both the normative, which were emphasized by the functionalists, and especially the cognitive elements. As already discussed, the power of professions is based on their control of belief systems. They claim authority on the basis of their willingness and ability to cope with specified ills, issues, problems. They stand ready to diagnose conditions, to make decisions, and to take actions in situations in which others are—by presumption or by definition—incapable of action.

Thus to explain why organizations incorporate professional actors and belief systems into their own structures, we should not too quickly conclude, following a crude power interpretation, that they do so only because professionals have created a monopoly based on the power of the state, which requires employers to use only certified practitioners (although such arrangements certainly exist in many cases). (See, for example, Freidson, 1986, pp. 71-73.) Although elements of coercion may be involved, the situation is often more interesting and complex. An institutionalist view would suggest that organizations willingly incorporate professionals (just as an individual client may voluntarily call in a professional practitioner) because they can be expected to absorb or reduce uncertainty for their employer, making decisions and handling problems in ways widely viewed as acceptable and legitimate (Meyer and Rowan, 1977). Employing professionals constitutes a solution not necessarily because the resulting outcome is successful but because, as Larson (1977, p. 198) argues, bringing in a professional "makes the use of discretion predictable. It relieves bureaucratic organizations of responsibility for devising their own mechanisms of control in the discretionary areas of work. There need be no basic conflict between the professional expectation of autonomy at work and large-scale bureaucratic organizations which create, by their technology, areas of discretion."

Institutional controls, such as those exercised by professional occupations, are sometimes built into organizational structures but may also bypass them, placing constraints on the activities of organizational participants in the absence of specific hierarchical controls or visible sanctions. Thus, professional controls can operate in the absence of explicit organizational controls (Scott, 1987a, pp. 506-507).

Throughout much of the period under review, sociological analysts of medical care have insisted on the relative efficacy and importance of "direct" social controls based on visibility of work, assessments of performance, and meaningful sanctions (Dornbusch and Scott, 1975; Freidson, 1975). Organizational controls—such as those exercised within group-practice clinics or health maintenance organizations—are asserted to be superior to institutional controls.

By contrast, the institutional perspective reminds us of the reality and power of symbolic controls. A remarkable feature of cognitive controls is their often unobtrusive nature: Cognitive models, when dominant, are virtually invisible. They rest on taken-for-granted beliefs and assumptions. They exercise control in the absence of visible sanctions; control resides in the cultural systems, not in the structural frameworks.

Such conceptions, in our view, move us toward capturing the distinctive features of professional actors. These explanations are not inconsistent with power interpretations; rather, they greatly expand the meaning of power, and they greatly enlarge the mechanisms by means of which power is acquired and exercised. Mann (1986) refers to such power as *ideological power* and includes among its hallmarks "transcendence" and "diffuseness." In ways we have just illustrated, ideological power is "sociospatially transcendent," spanning and interpenetrating the more conventional, "secular" sources of organizational authority. And, unlike bureaucratic power, it is not concentrated among a subset of participants but diffused throughout the population of practitioners (Mann, 1986, pp. 8, 23).

Connecting Institutional and Technical Aspects of Environments. Meyer and Scott (1983; Scott, 1987b) have argued that it is useful to distinguish two facets of organizational environments: institutional and technical. Institutional environments are characterized by the elaboration of rules and requirements to which individual organizations must conform in order to receive legitimacy and support. Technical environments are those in which organizations are rewarded for effective and efficient performance. Institutional environments reward organizations that have correct structures and processes; technical environments reward organizations that achieve correct outcomes.

It is an error, however, to differentiate too sharply between institutional and technical elements. All environments contain both technical and institutional elements, but the strength of these forces varies greatly across sectors. The medical care sector seems to combine relatively strong institutional and technical forces (Scott, 1982a). Professions are well known for placing great emphasis on their processes and procedures; they are usually reluctant to have their evaluations based on the success of the outcomes they achieve. Still, those professions whose body of practice rests on a scientific base are under pressure to take outcomes into account, to use them as the basis for selecting among procedures and improving practice. These pressures come from within the professions as well as from outside.

Internal groups emphasizing outcomes include a diverse collection of actors: basic research scientists, clinical researchers in medical settings, medical educators, medical care researchers, and pathologists. Reform-oriented physicians are especially likely to cluster in tertiary-care medical centers or to be found in major research units such as the National Institutes of Health. These individuals and groups provide information to external reform constituencies and form alliances with them.

External groups pressing for increased emphasis on outcome evaluations include many consumer-advocacy groups, insurance companies, employers who provide health care benefits, and government agencies regulating health care activities. Manufacturers of pharmaceuticals and of new health care technologies press for the introduction of their innovations. As noted, coalitions often develop that link internal (professional) and external advocates of change and reform. Alford (1975) refers to this diverse coalition of interests as "health care rationalizers." Largely because of the efforts of this coalition, technical developments and criteria shape institutional structures in the medical care sector.

But influence flows in both directions: Technical processes focus on outcomes, but institutional beliefs determine which types or aspects of outcomes are to be pursued. Thus the medical profession in the United States has made prolonging life the preeminent outcome. Alternatives such as relief of pain or maximizing functional status have less priority. Such value choices are deeply embedded in the institutional belief system. They are so fundamental that they are unconsciously accepted—taken for granted as part of the order of things. When they are challenged, as in disputes over euthanasia, passions run high, signifying that sacred beliefs are at issue. Every technical system is bounded by institutional beliefs and rests on such a foundation.

LOOKING FORWARD: ETHICS AS A NEW TOPIC FOR INSTITUTIONAL THEORY

In the first part of this chapter we chronicled how various strands of sociological work on professions and on organizations contributed to the development of the institutional perspective. Studies of physicians, other professional providers, and hospitals have been a particularly important source of illumination for the development of institutional theory. As a consequence, we believe that institutionalists now possess a significant body of conceptual tools to help account for many of the recent changes in the medical care sector. Up to this time, however, these tools have not been employed to address a topic that is of growing significance: the ethical dilemmas that have accompanied many recent changes and innovations. This neglect is a bit surprising in that many of these dilemmas appear to stem from shifts in the organizational arrangements for providing or paying for medical care.

Increased Interest in Medical Ethics

Medical care in the United States has always been accompanied by discourse on its ethical premises (Starr, 1982), but such discussion became particularly prevalent in the 1980s (Gray, forthcoming). The number of symposia, printed materials, and conferences on bioethics, medical-research ethics, and the ethics of health care delivery held or produced since 1980 is simply staggering. The timing of this increased interest—at least among academics—can be inferred from the starting dates of professional journals on medical ethics. The medical library at Harvard currently subscribes to eighteen journals on medical ethics. Of these, none was in existence prior to 1970, one developed prior to 1975, five emerged between 1975 and 1980, and twelve were founded since 1980.

An examination of the content of the discourse on medical ethics suggests its links to the organization of medical care. As these organizational arrangements have been undergoing rapid change, attention to ethical issues has increased.

Most discussions of medical ethics can be categorized into one of three types. The first, and most sensational, category is ethical concerns that accompany the development of new medical technologies. Fetal termination, in vitro fertilization, life-support technologies, organ transplants, and growth hormones are just a few examples of new technologies that have stirred up significant public and scholarly debate on ethical issues. These technologies push the issue of what is life and raise questions about what limits, if any, should be placed on medical intervention. Certainly, the speed and sheer magnitude of recent medical innovation explain in part the dramatic increase in attention to medical ethics.

We believe, however, that the organizational changes that have accompanied medical innovations are also important in accounting for the escalation in ethical concerns. Most innovations are produced by pharmaceutical, medical-equipment, and biotechnology firms that are governed by commercial considerations and are driven by competitive pressures. There is reasonable concern as

to whether these conditions lead to cost-effective and socially productive innovations. More important is the changing role of government in fostering medical innovation. The federal government
has become the primary source of funding for the increasingly expensive research required for medical innovations; and it is the
primary source of payment for the new and, sometimes, improved
services that result from these innovations. In addition to the complexity of having a third party, governmental involvement intro-
duces new ingredients to decisions about producing and adopting
innovations—concerns about scarce resources, appropriate use of
public funds, safeguards, distributional inequities.

The other two categories of discourse on medical ethics are
even more directly related than the first to changes in the organizational landscape. The second category includes ethical issues related to organizational changes within the hospital sector, such as
the rise of investor-owned hospitals, the growth of hospital chains,
and changes in the structure of religious sponsorship of hospitals.
The third category of ethical issues focuses on recent changes in the
organization of professional practice, such as the growth of group
practice among physicians, the increase in salaried physicians, increased entrepreneurial activity among physicians, the emergence of
health maintenance organizations and preferred provider organizations, and the changing roles and responsibilities of ancillary professional occupations.

The introduction into the medical care arena of new organizational forms and different occupational groups and organizational arrangements elevates ethical issues to the public forum.
Differences among individual actors and organizations become formalized and, as a consequence, are likely to become the subject of
public attention. As Scott (1985, p. 120-121) points out: "Many of
the conflicts are not about new issues, but rather represent a new
decisional division of labor around old issues. Conflicting premises
contained in such decisions as whom to treat and how much treatment to provide are no longer buried in the inconsistencies of the
physician's role but are more explicitly subdivided and allocated to
different actors. What were role conflicts become organized, formalized, articulated conflicts."

The entrance of public organizations into the scene is especially pertinent here. Such organizations, particularly in the United States, are expected to allow maximum access to multiple constituencies and interests, dispensing information, providing opportunities for participation, and taking into account multiple viewpoints.

Treatment of Ethics in the Literature on Organizations

Given that many of the sources of the increased discourse on medical ethics may be organizational, it would seem natural to look to the organizational literature for help in understanding ethical dilemmas in health care. But explicit attention to ethics is rare in scholarly writings on organizations. Some consideration of ethical issues by practitioners and applied researchers occurs within specific organizational domains—such as business, education, and law—but little research has reached across organizational domains, and virtually no attention has been given to ethics in the general, theoretical literature. (For exceptions, see Kram, Yeager, and Reed, 1989; and Yeager and Kram, forthcoming; some consideration of ethical issues also occurs in discussions of organizational "pathologies"—see, for example, Scott, 1987b, Chap. 12.)

Although the recent organizational literature gives little explicit attention to ethics, implicit attention was accorded to these issues before the 1970s. Ethics are inevitably involved when researchers focus on organizational goals. Goals were a central issue in the foundation works of the field of organizational sociology. Weber's ([1924] 1947) essay on bureaucracy was concerned with how a cultural emphasis on rationality—in contrast to other possible goals—led to the development of a new organizational form. And Michels's ([1915] 1949) treatise on oligarchy in political parties chronicled how the original goals of participants were transformed by pervasive internal and external organizational processes.

The early organizational sociologists in the United States working within the functionalist paradigm also gave high priority to organizational goals. Goals, goal setting, and the importance of normative constraints were central themes in Parsons's (1960) analyses of organizations. Selznick's (1949) classic study of the Tennessee Valley Authority stimulated a series of important case studies pursuing Michels's thesis of the inevitable subversion of organizational goals (see also, Lipset, Trow, and Coleman, 1956). Simon's (1945) early work on administrative systems within organizations dealt explicitly with the value premises that underlie decision making. And Blau and Scott's (1962) well-known typology of organizations emphasized organizational goals by focusing attention on the question *Cui bono?* Who benefits from the existence and operation of the organization?

Attention to variations in organizational goals, and to the values and value conflicts underlying goal selection, disappeared in large part with the rejection of functionalism. Organizational researchers tended to assume the existence of some broad organizational goals—such as efficiency, effectiveness, survival, or, in the case of the Marxist perspective, class domination—and then concentrated attention on variations in the structural arrangements by which goals are achieved. Much empirical attention was given during this period to examining the ways in which technological factors and environmental forces influenced the structure of organizations, with little concern for the effects of these processes on goal definition or goal attainment.

As we argued in the first part of this chapter, however, the institutional approach has revived interest in the symbolic aspects of organizations, including the ways in which organizational values are shaped by both the definition of organizational goals and the strategies employed in their pursuit.

An Institutional Approach to Organizational Ethics: Some Preliminary Thoughts

The development of an institutional approach to the study of organizational ethics is beyond the scope of this chapter. Instead, we offer some early, preliminary thoughts about how such an approach might differ from previous treatments of ethical disputes. For illustrative purpose, we use Simon's (1945) well-known organizational decision-making model as a point of comparison. (See also March and Simon, 1958; Simon, 1964.)

As we noted previously, the topic of organizational ethics has been treated implicitly by theorists under the guise of analyzing the values and norms that underlie organizational goals. Simon's model of decision making emphasizes this attachment of ethical considerations to organizational goals. According to Simon, an organization controls activity within its boundaries by creating a hierarchy of desired ends and then specifying limiting directives about the means to be used to achieve each desired end. Value premises— premises about what is morally or materially desirable—underlie decisions about ends, while factual premises—premises about how the world operates empirically—underlie decisions about means.

It follows from this distinction that choices of ends cannot be invalidated empirically but that choices of means are subject to such invalidation. Ends can be evaluated only by their consistency with higher-level ends; and organizations seek rationality by creating links among means and ends—means-ends chains—such that each subgoal is designed to contribute to a general goal, or end. Simon also argues that as one moves down the ends-means chains, ends are increasingly constrained by ends-and-means decisions at higher levels. Thus, the value component of decisions concerning ends declines as one moves down the hierarchy.

An institutional perspective on how ethical values enter into organizational activities differs from Simon's analysis in three important ways. First, an institutional approach would insist that value premises underlie not only the selection of goals but also the choice of means in organizations. Decisions about means may initially be based on empirically guided criteria, but such means often over time become "infused with value beyond the technical requirements of the task at hand" (Selznick, 1957, p. 17).

The prevalence of fee-for-service payment in the medical sector is an example of a highly institutionalized means. Its adoption was a hard-won political victory for physicians; it freed them from any mediation in medical markets by public or private organizations (Starr, 1982, pp. 25–26, 323–325). But since its adoption it has become enshrined as a moral necessity. The moral rationale for fee-for-service payment is based on two assumptions. The first assumption is that physicians, who are bound to a fiduciary ethic, can put a patient's interests first only if they act solely as the agent of the patient. Fee-for-service is a mechanism that directly binds the physician as agent of the patient and hence prevents conflicts of interest that would enter if doctors were paid by other parties. The second assumption is that an unmediated payment system in which patients pay flat rates to physicians would lead to increased competition among physicians; such competition would be detrimental to patients because unscrupulous physicians could undercut ethical practitioners by offering lower rates and cutting back on the quality of care.

This line of moral construction protected the fee-for-service provision from serious attack until the 1970s, and still today it remains the most common method of payment for medical services in the United States, even though it creates incentives for the provision of unnecessary services and clearly inflates medical care costs. The central point, however, is that ethical concerns are closely tied in with the selection of means as well as ends—in this instance, with decisions about provisions for care and compensation for providers—and that as these arrangements undergo change, ethical discourse is fueled.

Second, an institutional perspective would also differ from Simon's conception of the sources of ethical rules. According to Simon, the validation of the ultimate ends and means selected by an organization is an internal affair. Organizational participants— in particular, top executives—make and are expected to justify the selection of organizational goals. From an institutional perspective, by contrast, organizations are viewed as importing many of their goals and the routines for achieving them from the environment. Validation of these cognitive systems—both ends and theories of practice—occurs in key arenas in the environment of organizations rather than within the organization. The nation-state, the professions, and extremely successful organizations that serve as moral models are three of the most important external sources of validated goals and legitimated means.

An awareness of the external sources of ethical models raises new questions about patterns in organizational ethics. For example, do different sources of ethical prescription for organizational actions endorse different types of organizational features? Professions tend toward ethical explanations that favor an exclusive focus on the needs of the client in treatment and the unrestricted rights of the practitioner to determine what those needs are, while governments tend toward ethical patterns that emphasize equal treatment for clients regarded as similar and hence support attempts to circumscribe discretion and increase formalization.

A related question is, How do organizations balance the demands associated with the ethical premises held by different institutional actors in their environments? The different moral demands of administrators and physicians have, historically, been partially accommodated by the bifurcated power structure of hospitals. But now we have a multitude of organized actors each embracing somewhat varying ethical imperatives. The modern landscape includes corporate headquarters of for-profit as well as nonprofit hospital systems; individual hospital administrations, which must accommodate both the concerns of their professional staffs and local community and constituency interests; third-party payers, whose varying plans and formulas express diverse value preferences; organized employer associations with an interest in curtailing or at least containing employee benefits; marketing divisions of drug and medical appliance manufacturers, which are interested in maximizing the sales and market shares of their products; governmental financial and regulatory agencies, whose interests range from equality of access to cost containment to encouraging new scientific breakthroughs.

As the number and variety of organizational agents pursuing specific values and goals in a boundedly rational manner increase, so do explicit conflicts over ethical priorities and so does the babble of ethical discourse. And, as Scott (1985: 121) notes: "The issues and participants increasingly transcend the boundaries of individual medical care organizations. Individual participants such as Alain Enthoven and Michael DeBakey and collective actors such as the Institute of Medicine and the Health Care Financing Administration conduct their debates in the halls of Congress and the pages of the New York Times."

The question of how the ethical premises of organizations undergo change is the third area in which we think an institutional perspective on organizational ethics would develop alternatives to previous approaches. According to Simon—and also Selznick (1957)—organizational elites select the value premises undergirding organizational goals. This argument implies that such elites are relatively free to change their organization's value premises or mission if they are so inclined. However, an institutional perspective would argue that organizational elites have little latitude to change the value premises of their organizations because they are bound by environmental definitions of moral activity. In general, organizational ethics are conservative, for it is difficult to change arrangements and activities that are infused with moral worth.

Nevertheless, major shifts in organizational fields can and do occur, as is demonstrated by recent changes in the medical care sector. We believe that institutional theorists, who are, by their own admission, weak in explaining (not to mention, predicting) changes in institutional environments (DiMaggio, 1988; Zucker, 1988), have much to learn by paying close attention to such transformations, especially those, like the rise of investor-owned hospitals, that violate existing moral doctrines within an organizational domain.

Conclusion

This chapter has examined the historical interplay between sociological studies of the medical care sector and the development of organizational theory. We believe that the institutional perspective has evolved in part as a promising product of that interplay. Research in the medical care sector has informed institutional theory because professional forms are stronger and their influence clearer in this arena than in many others. Here too, we have seen nation-states—even the relatively passive American version—take an active role in both supporting and constraining the sector's competing groups and movements. And, more than in many other sectors, we can observe here the strong interplay of technical and institutional forces.

Still, much work needs to be done if this new perspective is to benefit fully from the knowledge that has been generated by medical care researchers. Specifically, we have suggested that the discourse on medical ethics that emerged during the 1980s might constitute a strategic topic for organizational theorists interested in reasserting the importance of cultural values as factors affecting organizational structures, activities, and change. We hope that as we move "forward to the future," this issue will receive increased attention.

References

Abbott, A. *The System of Professions: An Essay on the Division of Expert Labor.* Chicago: University of Chicago Press, 1988.

Alexander, J. A., and Amburgey, T. L. "The Dynamics of Change in the American Hospital Industry: Transformation or Selection?" *Medical Care Review*, 1987, *44*, 279–321.

Alexander, J. A., and Scott, W. R. "The Impact of Regulation on the Administrative Structure of Hospitals." *Hospital and Health Services Administration*, 1984, *29*, 71–85.

Alford, R. R. *Health Care Politics: Ideological and Interest Group Barriers to Reform.* Chicago: University of Chicago Press, 1975.

Bankston, M. *Organizational Reporting in a School District: State and Federal Programs.* Project Report 82-A10. Stanford, Calif.: Institute for Research on Finance and Governance, Stanford University, 1982.

Ben-David, J. "Professions in the Class Systems of Present-Day Societies." *Current Sociology*, 1963–1964, *12*, 247–330.

Bennis, W. G., Berkowitz, N., Affinito, M., and Malone, M. "Reference Groups and Loyalties in the Out-Patient Department." *Administrative Science Quarterly*, 1958, *2*, 481–500.

Berlant, J. *Profession and Monopoly: A Study of Medicine in the United States and Great Britain.* Berkeley: University of California Press, 1975.

Blau, P. M., and Scott, W. R. *Formal Organizations: A Comparative Approach.* San Francisco: Chandler, 1962.

Bledstein, B. J. *The Culture of Professionalism.* New York: Norton, 1976.

Bucher, R., and Strauss, A. "Professions in Process." *American Journal of Sociology*, 1961, *66*, 325–334.

Caplow, T. *The Sociology of Work.* Minneapolis: University of Minnesota Press, 1954.

Carr-Saunders, A. M., and Wilson, P. A. *The Professions.* Oxford, England: Oxford University Press, 1933.

Child, J., and Fulk, J. "Maintenance of Occupational Control: The Case of Professions." *Work and Occupations,* 1982, *9,* 155–192.

Clark, B. R. *The Higher Education System: Academic Organization in Cross-National Perspective.* Berkeley: University of California Press, 1983.

Collins, R. *The Credential Society: An Historical Sociology of Education and Stratification.* Orlando, Fla.: Academic Press, 1979.

D'Aunno, T. A., and Sutton, R. I. "Organizational Isomorphism and External Support in Conflicting Institutional Environments." Paper presented at a conference on "Advancing Institutional Theory," University of Michigan, Ann Arbor, June 1989.

DiMaggio, P. J. "Cultural Entrepreneurship in Nineteenth Century Boston: The Creation of an Organizational Base for High Culture in America." *Media, Culture and Society,* 1982, *4,* 33–50.

DiMaggio, P. J. "Interest and Agency in Institutional Theory." In L. G. Zucker (ed.), *Institutional Patterns and Organizations: Culture and Environment.* Cambridge, Mass.: Ballinger, 1988.

DiMaggio, P. J., and Powell, W. W. "The Iron Cage Revisited: Institutional Isomorphism and Collective Rationality in Organizational Fields." *American Sociological Review,* 1983, *48,* 147–160.

Dornbusch, S. M., and Scott, W. R. *Evaluation and the Exercise of Authority: A Theory of Control Applied to Diverse Organizations.* San Francisco: Jossey-Bass, 1975.

Etzioni, A. (ed.). *The Semi-Professions and Their Organization.* New York: Free Press, 1969.

Fielding, A. G., and Portwood, D. "Professions and the State: Toward a Typology of Bureaucratic Professions." *Sociological Review,* 1980, *28,* 23–53.

Foley, H. A., and Sharfstein, S. S. *Madness and Government: Who Cares for the Mentally Ill?* Washington, D.C.: American Psychiatric Press, 1983.

Freidson, E. *Professional Dominance: The Social Structure of Medical Care.* Hawthorne, N.Y.: Aldine, 1970a.

Freidson, E. *Profession of Medicine: A Study of the Sociology of Applied Knowledge.* New York: Dodd, Mead, 1970b.

Freidson, E. "Professions and the Occupational Principle." In E.

Freidson (ed.), *The Professions and Their Prospects.* Beverly Hills, Calif.: Sage, 1973.

Freidson, E. *Doctoring Together: A Study of Professional Social Control.* New York: Elsevier Science, 1975.

Freidson, E. *Professional Powers: A Study of the Institutionalization of Formal Knowledge.* Chicago: University of Chicago Press, 1986.

Goode, W. J. "Community Within a Community: The Professions." *American Sociological Review,* 1957, *20,* 194-200.

Gouldner, A. W. "Cosmopolitans and Locals." *Administrative Science Quarterly,* 1957-1958, *2,* 281-306, 444-480.

Gray, B. H. (ed.). *For-Profit Enterprise in Health Care.* Washington, D.C.: National Academy Press, 1986.

Gray, B. H. *Profit, Corporate Change, and Accountability in American Health Care.* Cambridge, Mass.: Harvard University Press, forthcoming.

Greenwood, E. "Attributes of a Profession." *Social Work,* 1957, *2,* 45-55.

Hall, R. H. "Professionalization and Bureaucratization." *American Sociological Review,* 1968, *33,* 92-104.

Hall, R. H. "Interorganizational or Interpersonal Relationships: A Case of Mistaken Identity?" In W. R. Scott and B. L. Black (eds.), *The Organization of Mental Health Services: Societal and Community Systems.* Beverly Hills, Calif.: Sage, 1986.

Hughes, E. C. *Men and Their Work.* New York: Free Press, 1958.

Jackson, J. A. (ed.). *Professions and Professionalization.* Cambridge, England: Cambridge University Press, 1970.

Johnson, T. *The Professions and Power.* London: Macmillan, 1972.

Kornhauser, W. *Scientists in Industry: Conflict and Accommodation.* Berkeley: University of California Press, 1962.

Kram, K. E., Yeager, P. C., and Reed, G. E. "Decisions and Dilemmas: The Ethical Dimension in the Corporate Context." *Research in Corporate Social Performance and Policy,* 1989, *11,* 21-54.

Larson, M. S. *The Rise of Professionalism: A Sociological Analysis.* Berkeley: University of California Press, 1977.

Lipset, S. M., Trow, M. A., and Coleman, J. S. *Union Democracy.* New York: Free Press, 1956.

Mann, M. *The Sources of Social Power.* Vol. 1. New York: Cambridge University Press, 1986.

March, J. G., and Simon, H. A. *Organizations.* New York: Wiley, 1958.

Meyer, J. W. "Centralization of Funding and Control in Educational Governance." In J. W. Meyer and W. R. Scott (eds.), *Organizational Environments: Ritual and Rationality.* Beverly Hills, Calif.: Sage, 1983.

Meyer, J. W., Boli, J., and Thomas, G. M. "Ontology and Rationalization in the Western Cultural Account." In G. M. Thomas, J. W. Meyer, F. O. Ramirez, and J. Boli (eds.). *Institutional Structure: Constituting State, Society, and the Individual.* Beverly Hills, Calif.: Sage, 1987.

Meyer, J. W., and Rowan, B. "Institutionalized Organizations: Formal Structure as Myth and Ceremony." *American Journal of Sociology,* 1977, *83,* 340–363.

Meyer, J. W., and Scott, W. R. *Organizational Environments: Ritual and Rationality.* Beverly Hills, Calif.: Sage, 1983.

Meyer, J. W., Scott, W. R., and Strang, D. "Centralization, Fragmentation, and School District Complexity." *Administrative Science Quarterly,* 1987, *32,* 186–201.

Michels, R. *Political Parties.* (E. Paul and C. Paul, trans.). New York: Free Press, 1949. (Originally published 1915.)

Millerson, G. *The Qualifying Associations.* Boston: Routledge & Kegan Paul, 1964.

Parsons, T. "The Professions and Social Structure." *Social Forces,* 1939, *17,* 456–467.

Parsons, T. *Structure and Process in Modern Societies.* New York: Free Press, 1960.

Rueschmeyer, D. *Lawyers and Their Society.* Cambridge, Mass.: Harvard University Press, 1973.

Rushing, W. R. *The Psychiatric Professions: Power, Conflict and Adaptation in a Psychiatric Hospital Staff.* Chapel Hill: University of North Carolina Press, 1964.

Scott, W. R. "Reactions to Supervision in a Heteronomous Professional Organization." *Administrative Science Quarterly,* 1965, *10,* 65–81.

Scott, W. R. "Professionals in Bureaucracies—Areas of Conflict." In

H. M. Vollmer and D. L. Mills (eds.), *Professionalization*. Englewood Cliffs, N.J.: Prentice-Hall, 1966.

Scott, W. R. "Health Care Organizations in the 1980s: The Convergence of Public and Professional Control Systems." In A. W. Johnson, O. Grusky, and B. H. Raven (eds.), *Contemporary Health Services: Social Science Perspectives*. Boston: Auburn House, 1982a.

Scott, W. R. "Managing Professional Work: Three Models of Control for Health Organizations." *Health Services Research*, 1982b, *17*, 213–240.

Scott, W. R. "Conflicting Levels of Rationality: Regulators, Managers, and Professionals in the Medical Care Sector." *Journal of Health Administration Education*, 1985, *3*, (2), 113–131.

Scott, W. R. "The Adolescence of Institutional Theory: Problems and Potential for Organizational Analysis." *Administrative Science Quarterly*, 1987a, *32*, 493–512.

Scott, W. R. *Organizations: Rational, Natural, and Open Systems*. (2nd ed.) Englewood Cliffs, N.J.: Prentice-Hall, 1987b.

Scott, W. R., and Meyer, J. W. "The Organization of Societal Sectors." In J. W. Meyer and W. R. Scott (eds.), *Organizational Environments: Ritual and Rationality*. Beverly Hills, Calif.: Sage, 1983.

Selznick, P. *TVA and the Grass Roots*. Berkeley: University of California Press, 1949.

Selznick, P. *Leadership in Administration*. New York: Harper & Row, 1957.

Simon, H. A. *Administrative Behavior*. New York: Macmillan, 1945.

Simon, H. A. "On the Concept of Organizational Goal." *Administrative Science Quarterly*, 1964, *9*, 1–22.

Simon, W. H. "Legality, Bureaucracy, and Class in the Welfare System." *Yale Law Journal*, 1983, *92*, 1198–1269.

Smith, H. L. "Contingencies of Professional Differentiation." *American Journal of Sociology*, 1958, *63*, 410–414.

Stackhouse, A. *The Effects of State Centralization on Administrative and Macro-Technical Structure in Contemporary Secondary Schools*. Project Report 82-A24. Stanford, Calif.: Institute for Research on Educational Finance and Governance, Stanford University, 1982.

Starr, P. *The Social Transformation of American Medicine.* New York: Basic Books, 1982.

Stevens, R. *American Medicine and the Public Interest.* New Haven, Conn.: Yale University Press, 1971.

Streeck, W., and Schmitter, P. C. "Community, Market, State—and Associations? The Prospective Contribution of Interest Governance to Social Order." In W. Streeck and P. C. Schmitter (eds.), *Private Interest Government: Beyond Market and State.* Beverly Hills, Calif.: Sage, 1985.

Vollmer, H. M., and Mills, D. (eds.). *Professionalization.* Englewood Cliffs, N.J.: Prentice-Hall, 1966.

Weber, M. *The Theory of Social and Economic Organization.* (A. H. Henderson and T. Parsons, eds. and trans.). New York: Free Press, 1947. (Originally published 1924.)

Wilensky, H. L. *Intellectuals in Labor Unions.* New York: Free Press, 1956.

Wilensky, H. L. "The Professionalization of Everyone?" *American Journal of Sociology,* 1964, *70,* 137–158.

Yeager, P. C., and Kram, K. E. "Fielding Hot Topics in Cool Settings: The Study of Corporate Ethics." *Qualitative Sociology,* forthcoming.

Zucker, L. G. "Where Do Institutional Patterns Come From? Organizations as Actors in Social Systems." In L. G. Zucker (ed.), *Institutional Patterns and Organizations: Culture and Environment.* Cambridge, Mass.: Ballinger, 1988.

3

Transformation of Institutional Environments:

Perspectives on the Corporatization of U.S. Health Care

Jeffrey A. Alexander
Thomas A. D'Aunno

Fundamental changes in organizational forms, shifts in authority and control patterns, and increased emphasis on cost containment and sound business practices were recurring themes in the health-services literature in the 1980s. These writings document the transformation of a cottage industry, controlled largely by professional standards and norms, to a purportedly "rational" system guided by the principles of efficiency and cost containment. However, we have remarkably few theories that explain these changes and, therefore, their implications for current and future health-delivery practices.

In this chapter we focus on the corporatization of the health care sector and attempt to formulate some nascent arguments about the role of institutional theory in explaining this important change. It is not our purpose to apply existing institutional theory to the health care sector. Rather, we use the health care sector to raise fundamental questions about institutional theory itself, particularly its ability to address issues of environmental and organizational change. Specifically we ask: From what institutional basis has the health care sector developed? How is the institutional envi-

ronment of the health care sector changing? And what is the impact
of such change on health care organizations?

The second question has particular importance for the advancement of institutional theory. The institutional perspective has
not effectively accounted for the mechanisms of change in institutional environments. We maintain that strengthening these explanations is critical not only to the development of the theory per se
but also to its ability to distinguish itself from other, related perspectives (for example, resource dependence). Our focus permits us
to address the issue of the susceptibility of institutional beliefs,
norms, and cognitions to change and calls into question the permanence or transience of institutional systems. It also permits us to
speculate as to the processes by which institutional beliefs, norms,
and cognitions are changed. Finally, it allows us to look at the
health care sector as a hybrid environment, controlled by both technical and institutional forces. Such hybrid environments have been
largely ignored in institutional-theory literature and research but
are, as we will argue, subject to change dynamics that are fundamentally different from those of predominantly technical or predominantly institutional sectors.

Background

Starr (1982) has defined the corporatization of health care in the
United States as the penetration of the corporation into the voluntary health care sector and the extension of voluntary health care
organizations into for-profit activities. Clearly, corporatization has
multiple facets, among them: the decline in voluntarism and professional power in the health care sector; the introduction of new
organizational forms in this sector (multihospital systems, specialized delivery organizations, corporate restructuring and diversification); and the increased emphasis on running health care as a
business rather than as a social service, including not only increases
in business practices per se but also the adoption of symbols and
language associated with business. Cause and effect are difficult to
separate in discussions of increasing corporatization in the health
care sector. Indeed, much of the literature speaks of environmental

change as a somewhat amorphous array of events that encompasses both shifts in the environments and the consequences of those shifts. These changes are discussed at length elsewhere in this book but include a radical shift in the payment structure for hospitals from cost-based to prospective payment, a significant increase in the supply of physicians, the fragmentation of physician power and autonomy, shrinking capital markets, and rapid advances in technology. Furthermore, a reorientation in public policy from ensuring access to health care for the poor to containing health care costs has resulted in competition among health care providers for patients, physicians, and dollars (Alexander and Amburgey, 1987).

These and other shocks to the health care sector have introduced considerable turbulence and uncertainty into what once was a stable operating environment and have stimulated unanticipated but important changes in the organization of the delivery system. The traditional acute-care hospital is now facing competition from new, alternative delivery organizations such as health maintenance organizations, preferred provider organizations, and freestanding ambulatory-care centers. Links among hospitals and other types of delivery organizations have also emerged; they range from highly structured multihospital systems to more loosely coupled hospital consortia (Goldsmith, 1981; Zuckerman, 1979).

The distribution of organizational forms in the health care sector has shifted in this new environment. We have seen some redistribution in type of ownership—from the nonprofit, voluntary, freestanding hospital to for-profit companies that manage many hospitals (Gray, 1983; Pelman, 1980). Perhaps more pervasive are the changes within not-for-profit delivery organizations as they come to approximate the structures and practices of the corporate sector. We have witnessed the decline of freestanding health-care-delivery organizations and the rise of multi-institutional systems with the concomitant shift in the locus of control from community boards to regional and national health care corporations. Even hospitals that are not affected by horizontal consolidation are reorganizing through such mechanisms as corporate restructuring, a process that segments a hospital's assets and functions into separate corporations (Alexander, Morlock, and Gifford, 1988). Also in the ascendance are vertically integrated systems that enable health care organizations not only to provide acute care but also to embrace care preceding and following the acute phases of treatment (Conrad, Mick, Madden, and Hoare, 1988). Finally, and perhaps as a reflection of shifting patterns of institutional support, the rate of hospital closures has increased markedly. Approximately 350 hospitals either shut their doors or underwent a radical conversion from 1976 to the early 1980s (Mullner, Byre, Levy, and Kubal, 1982; Mullner, Byre, and Kubal, 1983).

Alternative Explanations of Organizational Change. Given the widespread and fundamental nature of these changes, how can one make sense of them? To date, open-systems studies of hospitals and other delivery organizations have addressed organizational change by focusing on "rational" strategic adaptation, a perspective emphasizing purposeful change to increase organizational efficiency or access to resources or both in the face of environmental contingencies. As Goodstein (1988) points out, this research suffers from several problems. First, it assumes that organizations will adapt to new environments without specifying the structure of the environmental conditions or the kind of adaptation organizations are likely to make. Second, much of the research is guided by resource-dependence theory (Thompson, 1967; Pfeffer and Salancik, 1978), which emphasizes horizontal relations and the individual organization as the unit of analysis at the expense of vertical linkages and properties of organizational sectors or fields. Third, little or no attention has been given to the role of the state or the professions in shaping change in the health care sector. Finally, and perhaps most telling, the research based on the rational-adaptation-strategic perspective has demonstrated only weak links between new organizational practices and forms and the outcomes of efficiency, effectiveness, resource acquisition, or increased market share. For example, Shortell (1988) assserts that multi-institutional systems have failed to fulfill the promises made for them in the late 1970s and early 1980s. Such disquieting evidence raises the possibility that the technical demands on health care organizations are not totally responsible for the widely discussed organizational changes.

We maintain that institutional theory provides the basis for developing an alternative perspective on the changes occurring in the health care sector. The institutional perspective asserts that organizations have normative as well as technical or structural sources. Organizations are created by and reflect the development and elaboration of institutional roles and beliefs that are independent of structural or relational complexities and of technical efficiencies. Such institutional roles and beliefs are often codified into "rational myths" (Scott, 1981; Meyer and Rowan, 1977). They are rational in the sense that they are represented in elaborated systems of laws, professional standards, and licensure or accreditation requirements that impute a means-ends relationship. They are myths in the sense that they cannot be empirically verified but are widely held to be true (and sometimes taken for granted). Institutional theories emphasize that the survival of organizations depends on their conformity to these externally imposed requirements. Conformity is expressed through isomorphism with those actors/agents in the external environment who are empowered to provide legitimacy and support to organizations "embedded" in the institutional system. Isomorphism is the process that compels one organization in a population to resemble others that face the same set of environmental conditions (DiMaggio and Powell, 1983).

At base, we maintain that a key to understanding changes in health care organizations is adequate conceptualization of the environment in which such organizations operate. As we will attempt to illustrate, this environment differs not only from the environment characterized by resource-dependence and strategic theorists but also from the purely institutional character of the environment described by most institutional theorists.

Institutional Versus Technical Environments. Meyer and his associates (Meyer and Rowan, 1977; Meyer and Scott, 1983) have differentiated two types of organizational environments: technical and institutional. Technical environments are those within which a product or service is provided and exchanged in a market. Organizations operating in technical environments are rewarded for effective control of the work process and are expected to concentrate attention on control and coordination of technical processes, buffering these processes from environmental disturbances.

Most manufacturing organizations function primarily in technical environments. Xerox and IBM, for example, allocate a large share of their resources to improving production methods, developing new products, using labor efficiently, and ensuring adequate coordination and control over their complex production, sales, and research activities. These efforts are aimed at increasing efficiency and productivity—outcomes that are rewarded in technical environments by increased profits and market share. Because of the importance of means of production to organizational survival in technical environments, Xerox and IBM also protect their production units from uncertain or disruptive environmental influence, including variable sources of raw materials and fluctuations in demand.

Institutional environments, by contrast, feature elaborate rules and requirements to which individual organizations must conform if they are to receive support and legitimacy. Attention is directed away from control and coordination of technical processes and toward conformity to externally defined requirements or regulations (Scott and Meyer, 1983). Public schools and welfare agencies are typical of organizations operating in strong institutional environments. Unlike technical environments, these environments do not recognize or reward effective or efficient production. Public schools do not receive direct support contingent on increasing the knowledge of their students. Instead, they are evaluated broadly on the basis of appropriate curriculum, certified teachers, and academic structure (grades 1–6) that conform to the external specifications of the school district or state board of education. The more institutionalized the environment of an organization, the more its structures and procedures are governed by external controls. This control requires specific arrangements in the organization that are independent of contributions to technical performance.

Technical and institutional environments thus have different bases for evaluation of success and tend to encompass different types of organizations. But they can occur together. Conversely, neither environmental condition may be highly developed. For example, mental health and drug-abuse-treatment organizations typically face environments that present neither strong demands for efficient production of services nor predominant belief systems to which conformity is essential (Meyer, 1986). Rather, these segments of the health care sector contain multiple groups that compete for influence and that often hold conflicting views about how treatment organizations should operate (D'Aunno and Sutton, 1989). Thus, we argue that mental health and drug-abuse-treatment organizations, discussed in more detail later, belong to a "hybrid cell" distinguished by a combination of relatively weak technical and institutional demands. (See Figure 3.1.)

Hospitals, by contrast, are located in yet another hybrid cell characterized by relatively strong technical and institutional environments. Although this environmental condition is unusual, other types of organizations find themselves in similar circumstances. For much of the twentieth century hospitals and other health care organizations have been subject to strong institutional pressures, including a broad array of governmental regulations and requirements. They are also influenced by numerous professional specifications that govern what types of personnel may be hired, how tasks

Figure 3.1. Organizational Types Associated with Varying Environmental Conditions.

| | | Institutional Environments | |
		Strong	Weak
Technical Environments	Strong	Hospitals Banks Defense contractors	Retail-goods manufacturers Research firms Information-processing services (software)
	Weak	Public schools Welfare agencies Religious bodies	Mental health organizations Shoe-repair shops Barber shops Restaurants

Source: Alexander, J. A., and Scott, W. R. "The Impact of Regulation on the Administrative Structure of Hospitals." *Hospital and Health Services Administration*, 1984, *29*, pp. 72-85. © 1984, Foundation of the American College of Healthcare Executives, Health Administration Press, Ann Arbor, Michigan.

are distributed among them, and what procedures must be followed in performing these tasks. At the same time, hospitals operate in a highly technical environment. Although they are not directly rewarded for high quality (for example, patients with better outcomes do not pay more for their care), patients and physicians make quality assessments that affect their decision to use one hospital in favor of another. The threat of malpractice suits and the required use of tissue committees and pathology reports are examples of other performance pressures. Also, more than most other areas of professional practice, such as law, education, and religion, medicine is influenced by scientific and technical developments in which efficacy can be verified. The technical requirements of modern medicine are considerable (for example, those of modern surgery) and often demand tight internal controls and careful coordination if performance is to be effective. Health care organizations also are being increasingly pressured to improve efficiency in the use of resources. Prospective payment systems, such as diagnosis related group (DRG) formulas, are an example of such pressure (Alexander and Scott, 1984).

Change in the Context of Institutional Theory. If we accept the thesis that the health care sector is subject to both institutional and technical pressures of varying intensity, the question becomes, How do organizations operating within such hybrid environments accommodate different environmental demands and how, if at all, do such environments change? To date, institutional theory has been relatively silent in both these areas. Scant attention in the institutional-theory literature has been paid to the situation of organizations that operate in environments characterized by both strong technical and institutional demands or by both weak technical and institutional demands. Most empirical studies have addressed the "pure case" of organizations that operate in strong institutional environments but face only weak technical demands (for example, public schools). Although such research strategies may successfully isolate institutional effects, it is questionable whether such organizations represent those that experience both strong technical and strong institutional pressures or represent neither. Furthermore, the few studies of organizations operating in hybrid environments have tended to suppress consideration of either technical or institutional demands. For example, institutional studies of the health care sector have focused on the organizational consequences of regulation or vertical links to funding sources or both but have largely ignored how those effects operate in conjunction with the technical demands of medical care (Fennell and Alexander, 1987; Goodstein, 1988).

The theoretical literature is somewhat more illuminating than empirical studies about the effects of institutional and technical pressures on organizations. Meyer, Scott, and Deal (1981), for example, hypothesize that organizations that function in sectors that are more highly developed both institutionally and technologically will develop more complex and elaborate administrative systems and will experience higher levels of internal conflict. Historically, we know this to be true about many organizations operating in the health care sector. Hospitals, for example, have typically operated with a "dual hierarchy of control," represented on the one hand by hospital administration and on the other by the hospital medical staff (Harris, 1977). These dual lines of control operate in parallel with each other but rarely have they intersected in such a way as to disrupt relative spheres of influence over issues related to control, resource allocation, and professional prerogatives (Scott, 1982; Alexander, Morrisey, and Shortell, 1986; Smith, 1955; Perrow, 1965). Administration in health care organizations has been effectively removed from the operational side of the organization (patient care). Through such dual control structures, the hospital's professional staff could attend to the requirements of the technical environment, while administration focused on satisfying the demands of the institutional environment. Although this dual hierarchy of control seems to have operated effectively (although not necessarily efficiently) for years, this system is clearly showing signs of strain (Alexander, Morrisey, and Shortell, 1986; Glandon and Morrisey, 1986). One might posit that many of the changes in the health care sector are, in fact, a reflection of the changing relationship between the institutional and technical demands in the health care sector.

The presence of conflict under conditions of strong institutional and technical pressures has been treated more extensively in the literature. Scott (1984), for example, has argued that the ascendance of managerial professionals has created a state of parity between clinical and managerial interests in health care organizations. This parity has manifested itself through the mapping of inconsistent and conflicting external requirements onto the internal structure of health-care-delivery organizations. The emphasis of managerial ideology on rational systems and cost-effective care has increasingly conflicted with the professional orientation of individual doctor/patient relations and the micro delivery of specific medical services. Conflicting claims to the "right way" to deliver health care, the presence of alternative rationalities for organizing work (professional versus managerial), and the inherent conflicts between technical and institutional pressures in the health care sector have, according to Scott, delegitimized health care organizations and have opened the way for competing organizational forms, particularly those that are symbolic of rationality in the American capitalistic system—private corporations.

Implicit in Scott's argument is the notion that the change in health care organizations is a function of change in the institutional environment of these organizations—the collection of rules and beliefs and relational networks that arise in the larger social context. These norms and beliefs are increasingly organized into systems of rules, meanings, and associations that link organizations with one another and with the wider social structures. Although this notion is now a common one within the institutional perspective, Scott departs from mainstream thinking insofar as he raises the possibility that changes in the institutional environment may be a source of delegitimacy for existing belief systems as well as a source of strength for new belief systems.

To appreciate this argument as a departure from "traditional" institutional theory we must first ask, What has institutional theory had to say about change? Some students of organizational theory would argue that the institutional perspective has simply ignored the notion of change, viewing institutional systems as sources of stability and inertia, and as catalysts for the regeneration of structures and processes in organizations (DiMaggio and Powell, 1983; DiMaggio, 1988). Empirical research using this perspective has focused on intrasector variation in institutional environments and its consequences for how organizations are structured. Implicit in these studies has been the assumption that change has been coincident with the development of the state, increased centralization of resource-allocation decisions, and integrated vertical systems. Several studies in the health care sector have examined regulatory structures across the states and their effects on hospital organizational structure and multi-institutional arrangements among health care organizations (Fennell and Alexander, 1987; Goodstein, 1988).

Other institutional theorists have focused more narrowly on change by addressing the question of how certain organizational forms are diffused within particular institutional sectors (Zucker, 1983; Tolbert and Zucker, 1983). These theorists are concerned with a fairly specific set of structural modifications (for example, civil service reform, educational reform) and assume that change within particular organizations is subsequently diffused in a wide organizational field. The rapidity and scope of change increase as these "innovations" are institutionalized.

Taken as a whole, however, institutional theory has not addressed change adequately in those sectors subject either to both strong institutional and technical environments (hospitals) or to both weak institutional and technical demands (mental health). Furthermore, when change has been considered, it is usually in the context of increasing state influence over a particular sector or innovation (Scott and Meyer, 1983; Alexander and Scott, 1984; Goodstein, 1988). The possibility of institutional entropy or deinstitutionalization as a process underlying change has been given little consideration. Finally, institutional theory has artificially constrained consideration of institutional dynamics to particular sectors or types of organization. We have few studies of cross-sector influence in precipitating changes in institutional structures.

Dynamics of Change in Institutional Environments

We argue that institutional environments, rather than having stable characteristics and placing consistent demands on organizations, are often in states of change and transition. Such changes may result from several processes, including changing societal values about efficiency in the production of goods and services, changing societal values about central authority, competition and political maneuvering among advocates of conflicting beliefs, and the failure of organizations to transmit their beliefs and values effectively. Transitions associated with these changes present organizations with distinctive demands. In turn, organizations may respond in a variety of ways, including using strategies to buffer themselves from external changes, adopting conflicting practices, changing peripheral practices rather than core practices, and manipulating the content of belief systems.

In this section, we discuss two types of changes in institutional environments: changes in the relative strength of technical (efficiency) and institutional demands on organizations and changes in the content of beliefs held by important groups in organizations' environments. We argue that these types of changes are distinct and carry different consequences for organizations. In other words, these two types of changes provide alternative explanations for the increasing corporatization of the health care sector, and they offer different predictions about the consequences of corporatization. Because of the inherent conflict, instability, and incomplete institutionalization that characterize hybrid sectors, these two types of change are particularly likely to occur in organizations presented with a combination of either strong technical and strong institutional demands or weak technical and weak institutional demands. Thus, our theoretical discussion is largely confined to those hybrid sectors, which have received little attention in institutional theory to date.

Changes in the Strength of Technical and Institutional Environments. Conceptual work (Meyer, Scott, and Deal, 1981; Alexander and Scott, 1984) has described how technical and institutional pressures of varying strength can combine to influence organizational structure and behavior. This work has not, however, addressed changes in the relative strength of environmental demands. Using Alexander and Scott's (1984) typology (see Table 3.1), several such changes are theoretically possible.

Of the possible combinations suggested by Table 3.1, those with the most complexity and interest involve simultaneous changes in the strength of both technical and institutional demands. To the extent that such changes occur, organizations must deal with a high degree of uncertainty. It can be argued, for example, that many hospitals are now experiencing a strengthening of their technical environments and a weakening of their institutional environments. For example, several states have made policy decisions to eliminate certificate-of-need programs (decreasing institutional constraints) in order to stimulate competition among health care providers (increasing technical demands).

A historical analysis of the health care sector provides additional examples that illustrate how changes can occur in the strength of institutional and technical environments. Starr's (1982) history of American medicine suggests that the content of both normative and cognitive structures in health care has been shaped by the dual traditions of professionalism and voluntarism. These traditions have not only been reflected in the larger institutional environment of health care organizations but have, in turn, determined the organizational structure and forms of hospitals, health insurance, and other medical care institutions. The medical profession benefited from state protection and political accommodation of its interests (for example, decentralized control over programmatic decision making, professional control over licensing requirements). Independent professionalism was the dominant norm in the health care sector until the latter part of this century. Structures and organizations maintained the integrity of the patient/physician relationship, freedom of choice in clinical decision making, and internal, rather than external, control of medical practice. Systems emerged around these notions to the point where they were considered by society at large and certainly by policymakers, regulators, and even managers as taken-for-granted conditions of effective medical practice.

Although some institutional theorists would argue that these normative structures eventually assume a life of their own and become codified in the political, regulatory, and professional requirements imposed on organizations, we raise the possibility that institutional systems, even though long-lasting, are not permanent or even stable. Indeed, institutional systems require constant "tending" to be maintained over the long term. In the case of the medical profession, internal cohesion and strong collective action were keys to this institutional-maintenance activity. The efforts of the American Medical Association, for example, were aimed at reinforcing the notion of professional autonomy in the face of the slightest cry for change.

The long tradition of voluntarism in American medicine has complemented the inculcation of professional norms into the institutional structure of the U.S. health care system. The notions of local control, community accountability, and philanthropic support of health care orgnizations have served to keep programmatic decision making from becoming overly centralized and at the same time have discouraged a cohesive, integrated health care system. The extent to which this tradition has been institutionalized is illustrated by the roles, power, and influence of hospital trustees. The literature suggests that these boards do little in the way of active management or policymaking in hospitals, and yet their existence "shows" the community that the hospital is indeed conforming to what society perceives as the best way to organize (voluntaristic control) (Pfeffer, 1972, 1973; Starkweather, 1988). Whereas trustee positions in the nineteenth and early twentieth centuries were critical for procuring external resources to support hospitals, this function has long atrophied in favor of third-party support and physician generation of hospital revenues. Yet having a board of trustees for a hospital has never been seriously questioned, and indeed, it is assumed to be an essential part of the hospital structure. If we accept the assumption that the profession of medicine and traditions of voluntarism have been responsible for the historical structure of organizations in the health care sector, the question then becomes, What has happened to those institutional structures to precipitate a change?

Literature on institutional theory is becoming relatively rich on the topic of the origins of institutional practices, norms, and structures. Meyer and Rowan (1977) emphasize the multiplicity and diversity of belief systems. The critical notion here is that no one belief system dominates and shapes the institutional environment of organizations. Rather, society has multiple belief systems that, in principle, may permeate sector boundaries and displace the dominant institutional culture within that sector. In a related vein, because institutional environments also vary over time, the structuration of any one societal sector is not static but changes as a function of changes in the institutional environment.

Zucker (1987) argues that if basic processes of social transmission are incomplete, the result is many partially institutionalized processes that lead directly to social entropy, a tendency toward disorganization in the social system. Except for a few highly institutionalized elements, the taken-for-granted conditions in the social system gradually erode. If this erosion is not continually countered by active intervention to maintain the institutional system, these conditions will become cultural artifacts and eventually will disappear. This argument suggests that institutionalization may vary not only over time but also in degree. We speculate that incomplete institutionalization occurs in those sectors where competing forms of rationality exist; in the medical care sector, for example, strong technical pressures operate on organizations in addition to institutional constraints.

These arguments give rise to the notion that institutional structures in the health care sector have, over time, undergone some degree of entropy and delegitimation. The technical requirements affecting the practice of medical care would, under these conditions, assume the dominant role in dictating the structure of health care organizations, and corporatization would simply represent the increased salience of technical requirements on health care delivery.

When technical forces supplant institutional pressures in the medical care sector, we will observe certain changes. As institutional legitimacy becomes less relevant for ensuring organizational survival, selection pressures on health care organizations will increase through market competition. Market forces and operating efficiency will determine organizational "success" rather than isomorphism with key institutional structures. Over time, there will be an increased number of organizational failures in the health care sector, as organizations that are less able to compete are selected out in favor of more fit organizations.

Institutional theory also suggests that administrative structures are only loosely coupled to production activity in those organizations that operate in predominantly institutional environments. This claim derives from the principle that organizational success in

institutional environments is based on conformity to externally imposed requirements and beliefs rather than on efficient production
of goods and services (Meyer and Rowan, 1977; Scott and Meyer,
1983). To gain legitimacy and support from the environment, organizations need to map onto their structures the structure of the
larger institutional environment. Thus, administrative structures
and activity are directed outward, toward the environmental actors
that provide such legitimacy and support. However, as technical
pressures in the environment gradually become salient, administrative elements in health care organizations will attend to buffering
the technical core from environmental disturbances and to coordination of medical care delivery by administrative units. Over time
then, we would expect to find increased control and coordination
by administrative units and an increase in mergers, consolidations,
and vertical integration as health care organizations attempt to
buffer or manage environmental threats and protect their technical
core from disturbances in that environment.

In sectors with strong institutional environments we find a
fair amount of structural homogeneity across organizations as they
attempt to map onto their own structures important characteristics
of the institutional environment. Hospitals, for example, more or
less resembled one another as they conformed to widely held beliefs
and requirements that legitimated them in the larger society. As
institutional norms and standards break down, however, and are
supplanted by demanding technical requirements, no longer will a
dominant set of institutional beliefs or requirements or both provide "structuration" in the medical care sector. In fact, there is no
one best way to organize in order to achieve technical efficiencies
and superior performance in the marketplace. Consequently, over
time we would expect to find a great deal more variation in organizational forms in the health care sector as organizations become
less concerned with mapping onto their own structures the characteristics of the institutional environment and more concerned with
achieving technical efficiencies and buffering their technical cores
from environmental disturbances.

Institutional environments promote little interdependence or
coordinated activity between administrative units of organizations.
For example, the office of community affairs of a hospital might

have little or nothing to do with the finance department. In effect, such units are each established to deal with specific aspects of the institutional environment (Meyer and Rowan, 1977; Alexander and Scott, 1984). Concern is primarily on conformity to institutional requirements rather than on coordination of the work process. As institutional pressures decline through delegitimation and other means, such loose coupling will gradually give way to tighter, more coordinated activity among administrative units and a less "baroque" set of structures in health delivery organizations. "Lean and mean" rather than elaborated and complex will describe these administrative structures.

We anticipate that all these changes will not be abrupt shifts in the health care sector but gradual transformations as institutional systems experience entropy and technical pressures gain ascendance. Indeed, these types of transitions will be prolonged, lasting many years, for two reasons. First, competition, concern for efficiency, and other technical demands themselves are socially constructed (Scott, 1984). The meaning of competition and efficiency for a particular sector or industry needs to evolve and come to be widely shared. Such a process requires time.

Second, organizations and their leaders are likely to resist such transitions because they create uncertainty and threaten organizational survival. Thus, we expect organizations to respond in part by lobbying and forming trade associations to defend traditional beliefs and values in the sector (D'Aunno and Zuckerman, 1987). Lobbying efforts at the state and federal level will appeal to the need to respect "traditional values" and maintain the status quo. Competitive pressures at the local level, however, will probably require significant changes in technical processes as well as the development of strategies such as diversification. Making efforts to buffer themselves against local competitors while also attempting to slow erosion of institutional protection will tax organizations and their leaders.

As the transition from institutional to technical dominance works itself out, the potential for conflict between the previously dominant institutionalized rationality and rising technical pressures is likely to increase. In the health care sector this might be manifested by professional (physician) political activity, increasing conflict between physicians and managers in hospitals, and the establishment of parallel organizations by those professionals committed to retaining their prerogatives.

Changes in the Content of Beliefs. Our second explanation of change in institutional environments is based not on shifts in the relative strength of technical and institutional demands but on changes in the content of the normative and cognitive belief systems that underlie institutional environments. A significant contribution of institutional theorists has been to emphasize the importance of beliefs and values in shaping organizational environments. We argue that belief systems change and sometimes undergo substantial transformations. Changes in the content of belief systems can occur in several ways. A useful approach to understanding such changes is to classify them along two dimensions: the extent to which new beliefs complement or compete with an established set of beliefs and the extent to which new beliefs originate within the sector or externally. Scott and Meyer (1983) define a sector as "a domain identified by similarity of service, product or function" that is related to but broader than an industry. Sectors include not only the focal organizations of interest (hospitals) but also the major organizations to which they relate, including organizations that contribute directly to or regulate their activities.

To understand changes in beliefs we will consider mental health and drug-abuse treatment. These segments of the health care sector, as noted, typically have been characterized by few technical demands and no predominant institutional belief system. In their early formulation of institutional theory, Meyer and Rowan (1977) recognized that societies often promulgate sharply inconsistent and conflicting beliefs. American society, in particular, is characterized by pluralism and value conflicts. As a result, in many sectors proponents of belief systems compete with each other for legitimacy, dominance, and the right or power to allocate resources. D'Aunno and Sutton (1989), for example, have examined conflicting beliefs about how to treat drug-abuse problems. Proponents of a psychosocial approach emphasize the importance of helping clients deal with the underlying problems that are thought to cause the abuse of alcohol or drugs. In sharp contrast, the highly influential Alcoholics Anonymous (AA) approach views drug abuse as a disease that can be cured only by abstinence. In the absence of compelling evidence about the superior effectiveness of either approach, proponents of both models continue to compete with each other for dominance in the treatment arena.

Success in such competition will depend in large part on the political skills of the actors and the congruence of their beliefs with the views of society at large. AA proponents, for example, have developed and disseminated emotionally compelling literature to support their beliefs. This literature began with *Alcoholics Anonymous* (known as the Big Book), which was written in 1939 by Bill Watson, one of AA's two founders. The Big Book has sold more than five million copies and its influence persists: About 800,000 copies were sold in 1986. Moreover, we appear to be in an era of conservative societal views that support AA's position on abstinence. Indeed, a prominent historian of drug abuse in the United States argues that we are entering a period of neoprohibition (Musto, 1988). Thus, we expect that AA's views on treating drug-abuse clients will continue to be widely held and will become the dominant beliefs in the field.

Regardless of the particular strategies and tactics used by advocates of various beliefs, transitions in beliefs are likely to have some distinctive features. Transitions in which dominant beliefs are being replaced by competing beliefs that originate within a sector will be relatively short in duration. Organizations will quickly adopt practices consistent with the new beliefs, even if to do so they must temporarily use conflicting practices. We base this argument on the assumption that rival beliefs within a sector typically are well known although not widely adopted. Furthermore, proponents of rival beliefs are probably familiar with the actors and channels of influence in a sector. These factors facilitate the diffusion of rival beliefs that become dominant. Nonetheless, in such a transition period, uncertainty will be relatively high for the organization's leaders, and they may play it safe by retaining traditional practices even as they adopt new ones, until the new actors are completely in power or hold positions of authority. Similarly, to the extent that dominant beliefs in a sector are being replaced by congruent beliefs, the transition period will be even shorter; organizations will not be compelled to adopt conflicting practices.

Mental health treatment in the United States provides a useful illustration of competition among rival belief systems within a sector. A variety of beliefs about how to treat mental health problems has existed for decades within the mental health sector (Grob, 1983). Prominent among these belief systems are psychiatric, or medical, models that emphasize residential care under the supervision of physicians and community models that focus on treating individuals in community settings using an array of professional and nonprofessional resources. In the early 1980s a community model (referred to as deinstitutionalization) gained wide support and in many instances replaced the psychiatric model. This shift resulted in the discharge of many inpatient clients to treatment in outpatient clinics. Consistent with our analysis, the shift from a psychiatric to a community-based model of treatment occurred in a few years. Indeed, opponents of the shift argued that it occurred too abruptly, with so little planning to meet clients' needs that they were "dumped" into the streets and became homeless.

The case in which dominant beliefs are replaced by competitors from another sector is more complex than the case in which competing beliefs come from the same sector. An example is the competition between the mental health sector (psychosocial model) and the drug-abuse-treatment sector (AA model) already described (D'Aunno and Sutton, 1989). We argue that the successful overthrow of a dominant belief system by an external competitor is difficult and occurs infrequently. External competitors not only must rely on their political skills and societal support but also must exploit weaknesses in their opponent's belief system. These conditions suggest that transition periods will be prolonged (lasting several years or more) and that organizations will respond slowly to pressures to adopt new, conflicting practices. Indeed, any conformity to new beliefs is likely to be only skin deep because organizations will initially adopt peripheral practices as opposed to changing their core practices and procedures. For example, mental health organizations that diversify to treat drug-abuse clients may adopt some AA language, and they may even hire some AA members who are familiar with AA's "twelve steps to recovery." But such organizations are not likely to abandon traditional mental health practices such as using psychological tests to diagnose clients' underlying problems (D'Aunno and Price, 1989).

The final situation we will consider occurs when proponents of a belief system transform the belief system themselves, either intentionally or unintentionally. Unintended changes in belief systems can occur for several reasons. First, proponents of belief systems can simply fail to transmit their beliefs effectively. Organizational leaders, for example, may fail to recruit and socialize new followers. As a result, long-term changes in beliefs occur because the beliefs are not passed on adequately from one generation to the next.

This kind of unintentional transformation in beliefs typically occurs slowly and may have the most prolonged transition period of any of the changes in institutional environments we have discussed. Slow, subtle changes in beliefs are likely to occur when there are no strong rivals to a belief system and, hence, proponents lose their vigilance in transmitting values effectively. The consequences of such changes are not likely to be substantial in the short run. In the long term, however, external groups may question changes in beliefs and practices. This kind of unintentional transformation in beliefs sometimes occurs, for example, in religious-sponsored hospitals that were founded by charismatic individuals. The mission of these hospitals was primarily to serve the poor, and they reflected a strong commitment to their founders' beliefs and practices. In some of these hospitals, however, these values were not effectively transmitted, and practices have changed so much that their not-for-profit tax status is called into question.

A second kind of unintended transformation in beliefs occurs as a result of failed attempts to expand the domain of phenomena or practices that a belief system "explains." D'Aunno and Sutton (1989) found, for example, that some mental health centers that diversified to treat drug-abuse clients began to adopt practices endorsed by AA and the drug-abuse-treatment sector. These mental health centers had held beliefs about drug-abuse treatment based on psychosocial models. But diversification as an organizational strategy resulted in the unexpected consequence of yielding to pressure from AA proponents. Furthermore, to the extent that they relied less on traditional mental health practices, these centers received less support from parent organizations and other sources in the mental health sector. In short, attempts to expand the domain of a sector and its beliefs can invite counterattacks. Efforts to respond to such pressure from proponents of rival belief systems lead to unintended changes in the beliefs and practices.

Intentional transformations in belief systems can occur in response to competitors or in response to changes in societal values or concerns. In other words, proponents of a belief system may recognize the need to alter their views in order to retain their legitimacy and dominance. Intentional transformations can occur slowly or abruptly depending on the needs of the actors involved. Sudden, severe external threats to dominance, for example, may cause proponents of belief systems to alter their beliefs quickly. Proponents will prefer, however, not to act quickly to alter public statements of beliefs because sudden changes can lead to crises of confidence and loss of legitimacy. In sum, belief systems are sometimes used in a chameleon-like way to protect organizations and their members. To meet expectations and to be viewed as legitimate by important groups, proponents of belief systems intentionally alter their beliefs.

Such changes in the beliefs and values held by hospitals are nicely illustrated in Stevens's (1982, 1989) work on the relationship of voluntary hospitals and the state. She argues that voluntary hospitals have shown remarkable survival and adaptive skills over the decades. As medical care has been transformed from charitable relief to the purchase of a commodity, voluntary hospitals have been able to present themselves, as political and economic exigencies arose, as private or public charities, as public utilities, or as businesses. In institutional terms, voluntary hospitals have presented themselves in such a way as to ensure a steady flow of resources and legitimacy from the social system in which they were embedded.

Stevens notes that recent writings about hospitals have presented voluntary institutions as private organizations that began as self-sufficient, endowed organizations. They have become inappropriately attuned to the competitive marketplace largely because of the economic and political insensitivities brought about through government regulation. The "return" of hospital and other medical care organizations to unregulated competition was a central motif for legislative bills of the 1980s, and the idea that hospitals are, have been, and ought to be regarded as businesses resonates through the hospital literature.

Stevens provides historical evidence to contradict this notion based largely on data related to a longstanding relationship between government and voluntary hospitals, a relationship that existed well before the Great Depression. Particularly salient in this analysis is her observation that the definitions of public and private have changed over time to suit the needs of the hospital industry and the medical sector. For example, the community hospital of the 1920s had ceased, in many respects, to operate as a charitable organization and had become much like a business. Hospital incomes rose rapidly between 1910 and the early 1920s largely because of increasing specialization, expansion of services and equipment, and the lure of the market for private patients. As private patients became the primary clientele for voluntary hospitals, the poor became the residual rather than the primary beneficiaries. Correspondingly, students of the hospital scene no longer described voluntary hospitals as public because they gave away care to the needy but because their capital was drawn from a combination of public sources, such as donations, gifts, bequests, and taxation (Rorem, 1982). As the older, nineteenth-century spirit of delegatory charity was overtaken by a stronger stance for government in the Progressive years, so the government's role was lessened in the market-oriented environment of the 1920s. These changes have resulted in concomitant changes in the meaning of public and private as applied to voluntary organizations and the presentation of the hospital organization as either private or public to promote its interests, if not its survival.

Stevens emphasizes the utility of ahistorical "myths" in legitimizing health care and health care organizations in the context of current ideological or political thought. Antigovernment theory, for example, rationalizes the appearance and strengthening of corporate enterprises, mobilizing democratic individualism on behalf of the corporation. Previously legitimate roles for the state in the provision of health care are easily jettisoned as a historical encumbrance as new institutional beliefs are carefully crafted. As institutional mechanisms, these ahistorical myths have a clearly defined utility; they are more than simply misunderstandings of fact based on insufficient information. Stevens characterizes these myths somewhat the same way institutional theorists might, as a combination of wish fulfillment and functional, crafted self-portraits of institutions and their ideologies adapted to particular times and circumstances. Indeed, she notes the value, as do many institutional theorists, of a commonly held language to signify apparently common beliefs in free enterprise, a right to health, competition, or whatever ideological beliefs are dominant. In sum, Stevens's analysis reinforces the notion that institutional systems do indeed experience transient states. In response, hospitals and other health care organizations are shown to be chameleon-like in their presentation of self, as their patterns of adaptation mirror the prevailing political, economic, and ideological environment. Critical to this process of institutional adaptation is the development of myths about the institutional history of the health care sector and the organizations operating in it. Revisions or distortions of history provide the new institutional "presentations" of organizations with the normative and cognitive foundations that they would otherwise lack. From this perspective, corporatization in the health care sector does not reflect organizational responses to increased demands for efficiency. Rather, corporatization reflects the conformity of hospitals to the belief that they should be businesslike. In other words, hospitals are simply creating and managing the impression that they are businesses that have the goal of increasing their efficiency and productivity.

The ambiguous status of voluntary hospitals as simultaneously both (and neither) public and private has been used to selective advantage in the past by hospitals as financial and ideological conditions have changed. However, the current trend toward identification with the private sector may be disadvantageous in the long run if the capacity for institutional adaptation to changing environmental circumstances is not maintained. For example, it may be the case that the more private the institutional posture, the greater the chances in the future of private sector/government confrontation.

In institutional terms, the risk of such identification lies in the inability of hospitals to adapt to new environmental circumstances once the new privatized identity, or organizational persona, has been institutionalized. This situation speaks to the issue of whether adaptation by organizations precludes adaptability. Current thinking on the subject suggests that change itself may be an institutionalized process, with those organizations required to change most often (for example, hospitals) finding it easier to change than organizations faced with infrequent environmental demands for change (Kurke, 1988; Hannan and Freeman, 1984).

If it is true that corporatization in health care is a response to changes in institutional beliefs, then there will be several distinct consequences for organizations in the health care sector. First, as organizations conform to beliefs about health care as a business, there will be increasing isomorphism in the sector. Health care organizations will come to resemble each other in form or structure. That common structure, however, will be markedly different from that characterizing hospitals and other health care organizations operating under the institutional aegis of the medical profession and local trusteeship. These new structures are likely to resemble those in the corporate sector—parent holding-company arrangements, multidivisional forms, and so forth. Similarly, organizational practices will become increasingly businesslike. For example, hospitals will adopt management-information systems not so much because they can be used to increase efficiency in producing services but because such systems create an image of a sophisticated business.

Second, as isomorphism increases, there will be a corresponding decrease in organizational failure as conformity is rewarded with legitimacy and societal support. Market forces or competition based on efficiency will not be strong enough to cause organizational failure.

Third, health care organizations will continue to have only loose control and coordination of the work process itself. Although they will present themselves as efficient businesses to meet the expectations of external groups, health care organizations will continue to allow professionals to work autonomously. Administrative procedures and structures established to meet external demands (for example, quality-assurance committees) will not be closely tied to the production of services.

In short, if the corporatization of health care reflects a change in the content of institutional beliefs, we can expect two general trends. First, organizations will conform to the belief that health care is a corporate, business enterprise. As a result, organizational structures and practices will differ markedly from those of the 1970s and earlier, when the prevailing belief was that health care was a voluntaristic, community, and professional activity. Second, health care organizations will, at least to some extent, be buffered from market forces or demands for efficiency because of the continued importance of institutional actors in providing legitimacy and support.

The consequences for organizations of intentionally conforming to changes in external beliefs are likely to vary depending on how abrupt and substantial such changes are. Less abrupt and less substantial changes in organizational beliefs and practices are typically easier to make because such changes face fewer inertial pressures (Hannan and Freeman, 1984). For organization members, abrupt and substantial changes in beliefs are particularly difficult because the power of values and ideals to motivate and to give meaning to work is eroded. However, less abrupt and less substantial changes in organizational practices may not satisfy external groups who value conformity to their beliefs. Thus, in intentionally conforming to changes in external beliefs, organizations are often caught between the need to meet external demands and their limited ability to do so.

It is important to emphasize that the view of organizational adaptation captured in Stevens's work and in our analysis argues that organizations not only are passive recipients of societal values and norms but also can respond aggressively by shaping beliefs about the value of their work. Furthermore, they can take steps to prevent changes in societal beliefs and values that would require organizational adaptation. In our view, there are three major ways that organizations influence institutional environments (see also Pfeffer and Salancik, 1978). First, organizations lobby local, state, and federal governments to influence formal rules and laws or to prevent the passage of legislation that could harm their interests. The American Hospital Association has been active in this regard. Second, organizations engage in marketing campaigns to influence public opinion and beliefs about their behavior. An example is the 1988 advertising campaign jointly sponsored by several health care associations including the American Hospital Association, the American Medical Association, and the American Federation of Hospital Systems. As part of this effort, full-page advertisements appeared in popular magazines (for example, *Time*) warning the public to "Defend the Home Front" by opposing cuts in the Medicare and Medicaid programs. Third, individual organizations or professionals join together to form trade or professional associations to engage in lobbying and marketing efforts. The American Federation of Hospital Systems, for example, was formed by for-profit hospitals to promote their interests. In sum, the perspective that organizations can shape institutional environments and demands has perhaps not been as well developed in previous work as it should be given the kinds of efforts just described.

Future Development of the Institutional Perspective

To the extent that the context of health care has evolved and continues to evolve from individual, patient/practitioner relationships to care provided by organizations, health care has become inextricably linked to its organizational context (Scott, 1983; Scott and Lammers, 1985). Organizational vehicles for medical-services delivery will continue to be a major focus of research. However, the rapid environmental shifts occurring in the health care sector and the unprecedented rate of the founding of new delivery forms require that change be a central concern of organizational research in the health care sector. We have argued in this chapter that institutional theory offers the potential for developing new insights into the corporatization of U.S. health care. However, the success of such efforts depend as much on the development of the theory itself as on its application to the health care sector.

This chapter has attempted to develop the general argument that the corporatization of health care in the United States has been precipitated by a transformation of institutional systems rather than by rational or strategic adaptation by individual organizations to changes in their operating environments. We have proposed alternative processes through which such institutional changes occur not to create theoretical ambiguity but to reinforce the notion that within the institutional perspective the process of environmental and organizational change is still in need of substantial development.

Our first theoretical scenario posits that corporatization in the health care sector is a function of the entropy of existing institutional systems and the ascendance of technical demands that have historically operated in conjunction with these systems. The second scenario argues that institutional forces are not weaker in the current environment but that the content of the belief systems on which they are based has changed radically.

Both scenarios rest on the premise that in hybrid environments institutional systems are unstable and thus more susceptible to change, entropy, and disruption. Another common element of the two scenarios is a shift away from the social definition of rationality in the health care system based on the norms and standards of the medical profession as supported by local, amateur trusteeship. In both scenarios, organizational change is a direct result of the weakening of professional standards and norms in the health care sector, along with changes in the attendant organizational structures that support, and indeed reflect, these standards. Whether the decline in professional "rationality" gives rise to increased technical pressures in the health care system or whether it results in the installation of new institutional beliefs modeled after those in the corporate sector is the primary question on which the two scenarios diverge.

Given that the U.S. health care system is still in a state of transition, it may be some time before the validity of these two explanations can be ascertained. However, the processes by which institutional systems change present a good opportunity for researchers in this area. For example, it is likely that political contests among competing interests will determine the reigning form of institutional structure in the medical care system (Scott, 1987). The political processes by which environmental agents attempt to lay claim to legitimacy in establishing the normative and cognitive foundations of institutional systems are in much need of further study.

With the fleshing out of the institutional perspective, it may also become clear that it does not obviate or duplicate resource-dependence or strategic-theory views of organizational change and structure. For example, the choice of strategic direction by a health care organization might be considered in the context of the wider systems of values, beliefs, and norms in which the organization is embedded. The institutional context of such changes has already been explored within the population-ecology framework to great advantage (see Singh and others, 1986). It has been shown, for example, that obtaining legitimation from key external organizations had a significant effect on decreasing the failure rates of voluntary organizations in Canada.

The discussion of environmental and organizational change in this chapter is only a first step in pushing the boundary of institutional theory beyond its current limits. Our formative arguments do not exhaust the range of possibilities offered by institutional theory to explain change in the health care sector. Other explanations—for example, those based on changes in the structural dimensions of institutional environments (fragmentation, centralization)—may be equally plausible and worth further attention. Other avenues of theoretical exploration might focus on the language, symbols, and rituals associated with life in health care organizations. As recently as the 1970s, for example, terms like *profit* and *market* were considered taboo in hospital circles. Anything remotely smacking of business practices was considered distasteful to the hospital and its various constituencies. The hospital administrator was just that, the head of a rather complex and somewhat disorganized not-for-profit voluntary service agency. Today a walk through any hospital would reveal some dramatic changes. Terms like *market share, product-line management, return on investment,* and even *competition* are now commonly used when referring to hospital operations. The hospital administrator title has given way to chief executive officer or corporate vice-president. The utility of these language and symbolic changes for the presentation of an organizational image is an area ripe for study.

References

Alexander, J. A., and Amburgey, T. L. "The Dynamics of Change in the American Hospital Industry: Transformation or Selection?" *Medical Care Review,* 1987, *44* (2) 279-321.

Alexander, J. A., Morlock, L., and Gifford, B. "The Effects of Corporate Restructuring on Hospital Policy Making." *Health Services Research*, 1988, *23* (2) 311–337.

Alexander, J. A., Morrisey, M. A., and Shortell, S. M. "Effects of Competition, Regulation, and Corporatization on Hospital-Physician Relationships." *Journal of Health and Social Behavior*, 1986, *27*, 220–235.

Alexander, J. A., and Scott, W. R. "The Impact of Regulation on the Administrative Structure of Hospitals." *Hospital and Health Services Administration*, 1984, *29*, 71–85.

Conrad, D. A., Mick, S. S., Madden, C. W., and Hoare, G. "Vertical Structures and Control in Health Care Markets: A Conceptual Framework and Empirical Review." *Medical Care Review*, 1988, *45* (1), 49–100.

D'Aunno, T. A. and Price, R. H. "Organizational Responses to Conflicting Institutional Environments." Unpublished manuscript, University of Michigan, 1989.

D'Aunno, T. A., and Sutton, R. I. "Isomorphism and External Support in Conflicting Institutional Environments: The Case of Drug Abuse Treatment Organizations." Unpublished manuscript, 1989.

D'Aunno, T. A., and Zuckerman, H. S. "A Life Cycle Model of Organizational Federations: The Case of Hospitals." *Academy of Management Review*, 1987, *12* (3), 534–545.

DiMaggio, P. J. "Interest and Agency in Institutional Theory." In L. G. Zucker (ed.), *Institutional Patterns and Organizations: Culture and Environment*. Cambridge, Mass.: Ballinger, 1988.

DiMaggio, P. J., and Powell, W. W. "The Iron Cage Revisited: Institutional Isomorphism and Collective Rationality in Organizational Fields." *American Sociological Review*, 1983, *48*, 147–160.

Fennell, M., and Alexander, J. A. "Organizational Boundary Spanning and Institutionalized Environments." *Academy of Management Journal*, 1987, *30*, 456–476.

Glandon, G. L., and Morrisey, M. A. "Redefining the Hospital-Physician Relationship Under Prospective Payment." *Inquiry*, 1986, *23*, 166–175.

Goldsmith, J. *Can Hospitals Survive? The New Competitive Health Care Market.* Homewood, Ill.: Dow Jones-Irwin, 1981.

Goodstein, J. "Institutional Change, Interorganizational Dynamics, and the Organizational Structure of the U.S. Health Care Sector." Unpublished dissertation, University of California, Berkeley, 1988.

Gray, B. H. (ed.). *The New Health Care for Profit.* Washington, D.C.: National Academy Press, 1983.

Grob, G. N. *Mental Illness and American Society, 1875-1940.* Princeton, N.J.: Princeton University Press, 1983.

Hannan, M. T., and Freeman, J. "Structural Inertia and Organizational Change." *American Sociological Review,* 1984, *49,* 149-164.

Harris, J. E. "The Internal Organization of Hospitals: Some Economic Implications." *Bell Journal of Economics,* 1977, *8,* 467-482.

Institute of Medicine. *For-Profit Enterprise in Health Care.* Washington, D.C.: National Academy Press, 1986.

Kurke, L. B. "Does Adaptation Preclude Adaptability?" In L. G. Zucker (ed.), *Institutional Patterns and Organizations: Culture and Environment.* Cambridge, Mass.: Ballinger, 1988.

Meyer, J. W. "Institutional and Organizational Rationalization in the Mental Health System." In W. R. Scott and B. L. Black (eds.), *The Organization of Mental Health Services.* Beverly Hills, Calif.: Sage, 1986.

Meyer J. W., and Rowan, B. "Institutionalized Organizations: Formal Structure as Myth and Ceremony." *American Journal of Sociology,* 1977, *83,* 340-363.

Meyer, J. W., and Scott, W. R. *Organizational Environments: Ritual and Rationality.* Beverly Hills, Calif.: Sage, 1983.

Meyer, J. W., Scott, W. R., and Deal, T. "Institutional and Technical Sources of Organizational Structure: Explaining the Structure of Educational Organizations." In H. Stein (ed.), *Organization in the Human Services: Cross Disciplinary Reflections.* Philadelphia: Temple University Press, 1981.

Mullner, R. M., Byre, C. S., and Kubal, J. D. "Hospital Closure in the United States, 1976-1980: A Descriptive Overview." *Health Services Research,* 1983, *18,* 437-450.

Mullner, R. M., Byre, C. S., Levy, P. S., and Kubal, J. D. "Closure

Among U.S. Community Hospitals, 1976-1980: A Descriptive and Predictive Model." *Medical Care*, 1982, *20*, 699-709.

Musto, D. F. *Historical Perspectives on Substance Abuse.* Ann Arbor: School of Public Health, University of Michigan, 1988.

Pelman, A. S. "The New Medical-Industrial Complex." *The New England Journal of Medicine*, 1980, *303*, 963-970.

Perrow, L. "Hospitals: Technology, Structure and Goals." In J. G. Mark (ed.), *Handbook of Organizations.* Skokie, Ill.: Rand McNally, 1965.

Pfeffer, J. "Size and Composition of Boards of Directors." *Administrative Science Quarterly*, 1972, *17*, 221-228.

Pfeffer, J. "Size, Composition and Function of Hospital Boards of Directors: A Study of Organization-Environment Linkage." *Administrative Science Quarterly*, 1973, *18*, 349-364.

Pfeffer, J., and Salancik, G. R. *The External Control of Organizations: A Resource Dependence Perspective.* New York: Harper & Row, 1978.

Rorem, C. R. *A Quest for Certainty: Essays on Health Care Economics 1930-1970.* Ann Arbor, Mich.: Health Administration Press, 1982.

Scott, W. R. "Developments in Organization Theory, 1960-1980." *American Behavioral Scientist*, 1981, *24* (3), 407-422.

Scott, W. R. "Managing Professional Work: Three Models of Control for Health Organizations." *Health Services Research*, 1982, *17*, 213-240.

Scott, W. R. "Health Care Organizations." In J. W. Meyer and W. R. Scott (eds.), *Organizational Environments: Ritual and Rationality.* Beverly Hills, Calif.: Sage, 1983.

Scott, W. R. "Conflicting Levels of Rationality: Regulators, Managers and Professionals in the Medical Care Sector." Unpublished manuscript, Stanford University, 1984.

Scott, W. R. "The Adolescence of Institutional Theory: Problems and Potential for Organizational Analysis." *Administrative Science Quarterly*, 1987, *32*, 493-512.

Scott, W. R., and Lammers, J. C. "Trends in Occupations and Organizations in the Medical Care and Mental Health Sectors." *Medical Care Review*, 1985, *42* (1), 37-76.

Scott, W. R. and Meyer, J. W. "The Organization of Societal Sectors." In J. W. Meyer and W. R.. Scott (eds.), *Organizational Environments: Ritual and Rationality*. Beverly Hills, Calif.: Sage, 1983.

Shortell, S. M. "The Evolution of Hospital Systems: Unfulfilled Promises and Self Fulfilling Prophesies." *Medical Care Review*, 1988, *45* (2), 177–214.

Singh, J. V., House, R. J., and Tucker, D. J. "Organizational Legitimacy and the Liability of Newness." *Administrative Science Quarterly*, 1986, *31*, 171–193.

Smith, H. L. "Two Lines of Authority Are One Too Many." *Modern Hospitals*, 1955, *84*, 59–64.

Starkweather, D. "Hospital Board Power." *Health Services Management Research*, 1988, *1*, 74–86.

Starr, P. *The Social Transformation of American Medicine*. New York: Basic Books, 1982.

Stevens, R. "A Poor Sort of Memory: Voluntary Hospitals and Government Before the Depression." *Milbank Memorial Fund Quarterly—Health and Society*, 1982, *60* (4), 551–584.

Stevens, R. *In Sickness and in Wealth: American Hospitals in the Twentieth Century*. New York: Basic Books, 1989.

Thompson, J. D. *Organizations in Action*. New York: McGraw-Hill, 1967.

Tolbert, P. S., and Zucker, L. G. "Institutional Sources of Change in Organizational Structure: The Diffusion of Civil Service Reform, 1880–1935." *Administrative Science Quarterly*, 1983, *28*, 22–39.

Zucker, L. G. "Organizations as Institutions." In S. B. Bacharach (ed.), *Advances in Organizational Theory and Research*. Vol. 2. Greenwich, Conn.: JAI, 1983.

Zucker, L. G. "Institutional Theories of Organizations." *Annual Review of Sociology* (Palo Alto, Calif.), 1987, *13*, 443–464.

Zucker, L. G. "Where Do Institutional Patterns Come From?" In L. G. Zucker (ed.), *Institutional Patterns and Organizations: Culture and Environment*. Cambridge, Mass.: Ballinger, 1987.

Zuckerman, H. S. "Multi-Institutional Systems: Their Promise and Performance." In L. E. Weeks (ed.), *Multi-Institutional Systems*. Chicago: Hospital Research and Educational Trust, 1979.

4

Emerging
Organizational Networks:
The Case of the Community
Clinical Oncology Program

Arnold D. Kaluzny

Joseph P. Morrissey

Martha M. McKinney

Health services are increasingly being delivered through new and diverse organizational forms. Whereas the health-services system once was populated by hospitals, health departments, and physicians with uneasy but predictable relationships, the present system is composed of a broad array of organizations and networks heretofore unknown within the health-services field. Cost-containment organizations, organ-procurement networks, and clinical cooperative groups are just a few of the new organizational forms that now constitute the health-services system.

These new types of organizations exhibit characteristics and raise issues that challenge existing organization theory. Increased interorganizational dependencies, multitiered administrative structures that transcend individual organizational entities, and rapidly changing approaches to communication and coordination require that theoretical models be extended or reformulated to reflect the realities of the current health care environment.

Note: The research on which this chapter is based was supported by an evaluation contract from the National Cancer Institute's Division of Cancer Prevention and Control.

86

The purpose of this chapter is to examine interorganizational exchanges and innovation-institutionalization processes with a community-based cancer-resesearch network known as the Community Clinical Oncology Program (CCOP). Experiences in implementing and institutionalizing this interorganizational innovation offer fresh insights into organization theory and suggest strategies for managing emergent organizational networks. Two specific theoretical perspectives are presented: an interaction model of interorganizational exchange and performance and an organizational perspective on innovation institutionalization. Although these theoretical models have different units of analysis, problem orientations, and explanatory propositions, they both focus on organizational learning and adaptation processes within the larger evolution of the interorganizational network (Kimberly, Miles, and associates, 1980). Each perspective highlights a different phase of the evolutionary process. The interaction model emphasizes key relational factors that affect network stability and performance, while the innovation perspective focuses on transition points between evolutionary stages—particularly the institutionalization of CCOP activities within participating hospitals and medical practices. Thus, the perspectives can be viewed as complementary rather than competing. Our purpose is not to present a detailed description of the theoretical approaches; this information is available from other sources (Hakansson, 1982a; Kaluzny and Hernandez, 1988). Instead, we assess the utility of the perspectives given the characteristics of CCOPs. We hope to demonstrate that these new organizational forms offer special opportunities to test the explanatory power of current organization theory and to extend it into new and exciting arenas.

The Community Clinical Oncology Program

The CCOP is designed to bring the benefits of treatment and cancer-control research to patients in local communities by enabling community physicians to enroll patients on clinical trials that previously were available only through major centers for cancer treatment and research (Kaluzny and others, 1989). As shown in Figure 4.1, the CCOP network consists of three major components: the individual

Figure 4.1. CCOP Organizational Relationships.

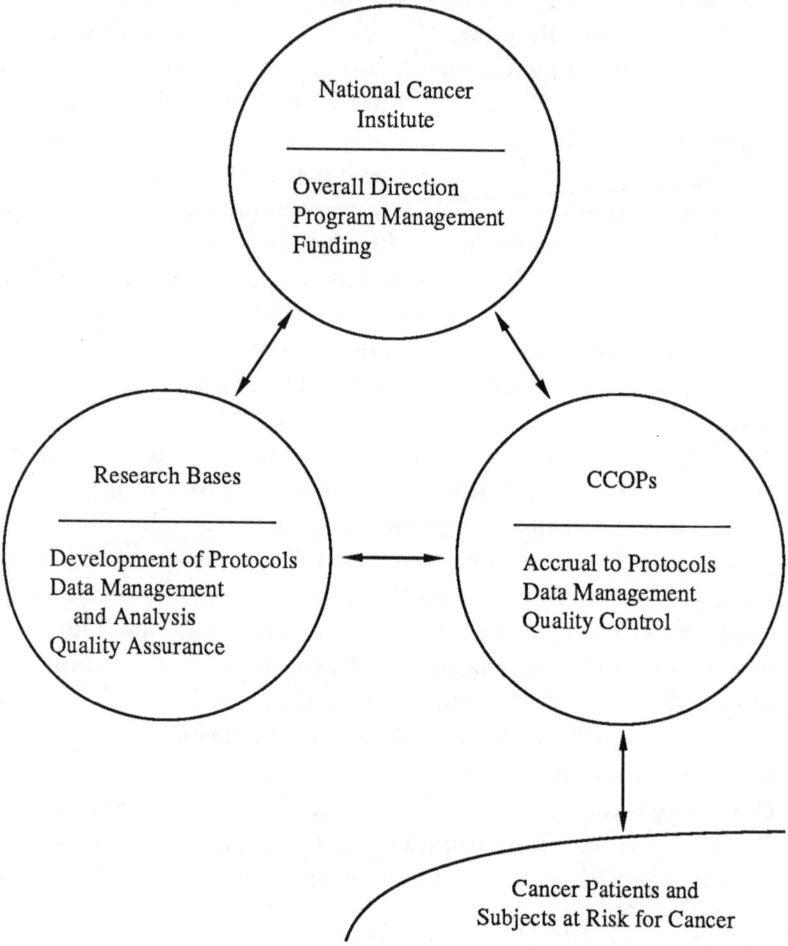

National Cancer
Institute

Overall Direction
Program Management
Funding

Research Bases

Development of Protocols
Data Management
and Analysis
Quality Assurance

CCOPs

Accrual to Protocols
Data Management
Quality Control

Cancer Patients and
Subjects at Risk for Cancer

Source: Leslie Ford, from a personal communication.

CCOPs, their designated research bases, and the National Cancer
Institute's (NCI) Division of Cancer Prevention and Control
(DCPC).

CCOPs are the organizational units that conduct research on
cancer treatment and control at the community level. They typically

consist of one or more community hospitals and a group of oncologists and other medical specialists who admit cancer patients to these hospitals. Although the hospitals may provide some financial and staff support, most of the administrative, data-management, and travel costs associated with entering patients in cancer-research studies are paid through cooperative agreements with NCI/DCPC. CCOP physicians register and randomize patients in clinical trials through the research base(s) with which the CCOP is affiliated. For each patient enrolled in a research-base protocol, the CCOP receives a certain amount of accrual credit. Because a typical assignment is one accrual credit per enrolled patient, CCOPs must enroll about fifty patients per year in cancer-treatment protocols to meet the NCI minimum requirement of fifty accrual credits.

Each CCOP is headed by a clinician–principal investigator or coinvestigators who are responsible for the management of CCOP activities. One or more data managers—usually nurses specializing in oncology—manage the flow of patient data between CCOP physicians and research bases and assist the physicians in identifying protocol-eligible patients. One of the incentives built into the CCOP cooperative agreements is support for physicians, data managers, and hospital support staff to attend research-base scientific meetings. These meetings provide opportunities for physicians and staff to learn about new research, participate in protocol design, and develop skills in clinical-trials management.

Research bases design the protocols for the treatment clinical trials and cancer-control research studies in which CCOPs and other research institutions participate. In this leadership role, they also collect, verify, and analyze study data; provide training in the management of clinical trials and cancer-control research; and monitor the patient enrollments and data quality of CCOPs and other research-base members. Research bases may be NCI-funded clinical cooperative groups, core-grant cancer centers, or state health departments. Each CCOP may affiliate with up to five eligible research bases, only one of which may be a national, multispecialty cooperative group.

DCPC is a constituent part of NCI, one of the National Institutes of Health. Through its Community Oncology and Rehabilitation Branch, DCPC establishes directions for the CCOP, provides funding to CCOPs and research bases, and monitors program progress. DCPC staff also work with NCI's Division of Cancer Treatment to review and approve proposed cancer-research protocols and to monitor the scientific value, quality, and provisions for patient safety of these studies.

Sixty-two CCOPs and thirty-one research bases participated in the first phase of the CCOP, which ran from September 1983 through August 1986. Because the focus of CCOP-I was on treatment-oriented research, selection of CCOPs was based on their potential to enroll a minimum of fifty patients per year in NCI-approved treatment clinical trials. An evaluation of the first three years concluded that CCOPs were effective in getting community patients enrolled in the clinical trials and that they met or exceeded all quality-control standards established by the research bases (Feigl and others, 1987). NCI records indicate that CCOP physicians entered 14,000 patients in clinical research protocols during CCOP-I.

In June 1987, after a nine-month funding extension, fifty-two CCOPs and seventeen research bases received three-year funding under CCOP-II cooperative agreements. Thirty-nine of the CCOPs and fourteen of the research bases had participated in CCOP-I, giving considerable continuity to the program. Although the CCOPs are spread over thirty states, they tend to be concentrated in the northeastern and north-central states, where almost 40 percent of the U.S. population resides.

Although the overall thrust of CCOP-II remains the same as that of CCOP-I, the new guidelines place major emphasis on cancer-control research in such areas as prevention, early detection, screening, patient management, and continuing care. To participate in CCOP-II, research bases must design and implement cancer-control research studies, and CCOPs must earn a specified number of accrual credits by entering patients in these studies. CCOP-II has five goals: to bring the advantages of treatment and other cancer-control research to individuals in their own communities by having practicing physicians and their patients participate in such research; to provide a basis for involving a wide segment of the community in cancer-control research and to investigate the impact of advances in cancer therapy and control in community medical practices; to increase the involvement of primary-care providers and other specialists (surgeons, urologists, gynecologists) with the CCOP investigators in treatment and other cancer-control research approved by NCI; to reduce cancer mortality by accelerating the transfer of newly developed technologies for prevention, detection, treatment, and continuing care; to facilitate wide community participation (including minority groups and underserved populations) in future treatment and other cancer-control research approved by NCI.

The inclusion of a specific requirement that CCOPs participate in cancer-control research and that research bases develop cancer-control research studies has increased the organizational complexity of both entities. Because cancer-control research is oriented more toward cancer prevention and education in healthy populations than toward the treatment of cancer patients, some CCOPs and research bases have resisted the cancer-control initiative. Others see the cancer-control requirement as an opportunity to develop a comprehensive program of research that links prevention, early detection, treatment, and continuing care. Although most research bases have organized cancer-control committees or modified their structures to facilitate the development of protocols for cancer-control research, the level of protocol development differs greatly from research base to research base. CCOP responses have ranged from minimal involvement in cancer-control research to the formation of local committees for cancer-control research and the active promotion of cancer prevention and screening activities within component hospitals.

The operations and institutionalization of the CCOP as a new organizational form can be only partially explained by existing organization theory. Succeeding sections of this chapter suggest ways in which extant theory can be modified, extended, and integrated to be relevant to the health-services and research networks that may well dominate the health care sector in the 1990s.

An Interaction Perspective on CCOP Performance

As a new organizational form, CCOPs must demonstrate their reliability and accountability to enhance their chances of survival (Hannan and Freeman, 1984). Patient accruals serve as the primary measure of CCOP performance because CCOP success in enrolling patients in clinical research protocols provides quick feedback on the effectiveness of new cancer therapies and enables more patients than in the past to receive state-of-the-art treatments in their own communities. Because CCOPs rely on NCI-supported research bases to design and manage the clinical trials, their accrual performance depends, to a great extent, on the quality and stability of the relationships that they establish with the research bases. An interaction model developed by a group of Scandinavian researchers to explain industrial marketing relationships in five European countries (Hakansson, 1982a) provides a useful conceptual framework for analyzing the effects of CCOP/research-base relationships on CCOP accrual performance. At the same time, certain characteristics of CCOP/research-base relationships raise issues and suggest links between variables that should increase the explanatory power of the model. A discussion of the interaction model and the refinements suggested by our study of cancer-research networks follows.

Basic Unit of Analysis. The interaction model draws on social-exchange theory and resource-dependence theory to analyze supplier/customer relationships and the factors influencing these relationships. Like social-exchange theory, the model emphasizes durable social relations between actors and adaptations that take place over time (Cook, 1987). Noting that stable relationships increase the efficiency of the exchange (Johanson and Wootz, 1986) and permit increased control over critical resources (Hagg and Wiedersheim-Paul, 1984), the model predicts that both parties will "invest" money, time, and talent in the development and maintenance of such relationships. Whereas social-exchange theory views dyadic exchange relations as "components of larger social structures of interest" (Cook and Emerson, 1984), the dyadic relationship between supplier and customer is the focal point of the interaction model. The objective is to understand the emergence, growth, and stabilization (or dissolution) of supplier/customer relationships by examining individual, organizational, and environmental influences as well as the interaction strategies of each corporate actor.

Application of the interaction model to CCOP/research-base relationships is complicated by the fact that research bases act both as "suppliers" of research protocols and "buyers" of information on how patients respond to different treatment regimens. CCOPs also assume dual roles as "buyers" of research protocols and "suppliers" of patient data. Although the interaction model does not consider the possibility of one organization's assuming both supplier and buyer roles, our interviews with CCOP and research-base investigators suggest that relationships are strongest when research bases emphasize the buyer role. This role downplays power differentials and focuses attention on improved productivity and data quality through trust and cooperation. One cooperative group chairperson summarized his group's relationships as follows: "We feel the success of our group has been primarily related to the cooperative spirit between CCOPs and the research base resulting from true mutual respect. Rather than treating our CCOPs as just case contributors, we have encouraged the assumption of leadership roles by the CCOPs themselves. We have sought out and respected their contribution to protocol objectives, protocol design, and protocol conduct. We believe that allowing such authority produces pride in the accomplishment of the group and provides strong stimulation for high quality productivity."

Problem Orientation. To date, most empirical research on the interaction model has examined the nature of customer/supplier relationships under different circumstances, provided examples of variations in these relationships, and attempted to explain the variations (Hakansson, 1982a). Although some investigators have moved beyond this descriptive research to assess how different exchange and adaptation processes affect the stability of customer/supplier relationships (Hallen, Johanson, and Mohamed, 1987; Johanson, 1988), the influence of interorganizational exchanges on one or both partners' performance remains largely unexplored. Exchanges in the form of protocols, patients, information, and power between CCOPs and their research bases provide a rich empirical base for analylzing how different types and levels of exchange affect each organization and, ultimately, CCOP accrual performance. Several hypotheses about these relationships are presented later in this section.

Key Concepts. The interaction model is based on four organizing concepts that require some elaboration to fit health-services
and research networks. The first of these concepts is resource dependence. The interaction model assumes that customer/supplier
exchanges are driven by a mutual need for critical resources. Under
NCI guidelines, CCOPs must affiliate with one or more research
bases to earn credits for patient enrollment. Although some alternative sources of protocols exist (for example, drug-company clinical trials), they are few in number and they do not qualify for
accrual credit. Thus, the patient enrollments that count for NCI
funding must take place through NCI-sponsored research bases.
The research bases, in turn, design randomized clinical trials that
require hundreds of patients in order to compare the efficacy of new
treatments with standard therapies. With many of these studies running simultaneously, they need CCOPs to help them recruit patients, administer the necessary treatments and tests, and evaluate
patient responses to the treatments. In addition, some research
bases, such as the North Central Cancer Treatment Group, rely
heavily on CCOPs to help them identify priority disease sites for
protocol development and to design protocols that are appropriate
for community settings.

Although the foregoing discussion suggests that the choice
of exchange partners can be strategic (Axelsson, 1987), the selection
process appears to be quite informal. In the words of one CCOP
principal investigator, "CCOPs seldom shop around for research
bases." They generally affiliate with research bases where their
physicians previously served as fellows, held medical staff appointments, or participated in a Cooperative Group Outreach Program
(an NCI-funded outreach program of certain clinical cooperative
groups through which community physicians can enter patients in
cancer-research protocols). These prior relationships reduce the perceived need for extensive search and create a sufficient level of as-
cribed trust to pursue an affiliation. The object is not to find the
"optimum" research-base affiliation but rather to find "suitable"
research bases with which the CCOP can develop a relationship
over a long period (Laage-Hellman, 1987).

Interactions are the second conceptual basis for the interaction model. Two types of interactions are necessary for maintaining

supplier/customer relationships. According to the model, short-term exchanges of protocols, patients, and information should lead to long-term adaptations in protocols, protocol-development processes, data-management procedures, and power-dependence relationships. Through ongoing interactions, decision makers on both sides learn each other's technologies, routines, and problems; modify their activities; and achieve a kind of balance in the relationship (Hakansson and Wootz, 1979; Hakansson and Johanson, 1988). Links become institutionalized into a set or roles that each party expects the other to perform (Hakansson, 1982a).

Our study of cancer-research networks suggests that adaptation may play a critical role in stabilizing CCOP/research-base relationships. When queried about the extent to which data-management and quality-control procedures had been adapted to integrate CCOPs into research-base activities, almost 60 percent of the research-base principal investigators reported high or moderately high adaptation (University of North Carolina, 1988). However, as Weick (1979) notes, adaptation may preclude future adaptive capacity if the two parties make too many relationship-specific investments. For example, a CCOP that develops data-management and quality-control procedures to accommodate one research base may find it difficult to modify these procedures when they want to work with other research bases.

In discussing supplier/customer exchange episodes, the interaction model gives only minimal attention to the ways in which different types of exchange influence each organization, adaptation, or performance outcomes. As Wilson and Mummalaneni (1986) note, the model offers the promise of fresh insights but, until the variables are linked, operationalized, and tested, researchers will not be able to assess its validity. Our preliminary analyses of qualitative and quantitative data from the CCOP-II evaluation suggest that the different types of exchange between CCOPs and their research bases are interrelated. Based on interviews with CCOP and research-base investigators, we have hypothesized that high information exchange, in the form of CCOP physician and support-staff attendance at research-base meetings and membership on scientific committees, will lead to patient enrollment in an increased number of protocols (increased protocol exchange). Moreover, we expect both these exchanges to precede sociopolitical exchange (defined here as CCOP appointments to committee and protocol chairpersonships).

In a cross-sectional analysis of the relationships between CCOP/research-base information exchanges, the average number of protocols used per research base, and patient accruals, we found a .61 correlation ($p \leq .0001$) between the number of CCOP physicians attending at least one research-base meeting annually and the number of patients enrolled in cancer-treatment protocols. The correlation between the number of CCOP physicians serving on at least one research-base committee and patient accruals was .48 ($p \leq .0004$); and the correlation between the average number of protocols used per research base and patient accruals was .42 ($p \leq .0021$). In addition, our research-base site visits suggest that the relationship between information exchange, protocol exchange, and CCOP accrual performance increases when the CCOP engages in sociopolitical exchange. One cooperative group spokesperson explained the moderating effect of sociopolitical exchange: "It has been our experience that accrual figures dramatically demonstrate a correlation with Group involvement. The more CCOP investigators are involved in protocol development and committee activity, the more patients are accrued."

Situational variables are the third organizing concept. The interaction model assumes that interactions between a supplier and a customer are "conditioned" by characteristics of the exchange, the interacting parties, the interaction environment, and the relationship atmosphere (Hakansson, 1987). By directing attention to these situational variables, the model offers more of an open-systems perspective on exchange relations than is traditionally provided by social-exchange theory. Thus, a CCOP's relationship with a particular research base can be analyzed by the types, amount, and direction of exchange; the size, funding levels, and organizational structures of both entities; the extent to which cancer-research funding is stable or dynamic; and the overall atmosphere of conflict/cooperation, closeness/distance, and trust/opportunism between the research base and its affiliated CCOPs.

Although the interaction model does not specify how these situational variables influence interorganizational relationships, our study of cancer-research networks suggests that the relationship atmosphere within a research base has a significant impact on CCOP performance. Interviews with CCOP and research-base representatives revealed radically different perceptions of the amount of CCOP influence within each research base, the extent to which CCOPs are encouraged to participate in scientific activities, and the areas of research that should be emphasized. One hypothesis guiding our research is that greater "psychic distance" (Hallen and Wiedersheim-Paul, 1984) between a research base and its affiliated CCOPs will be associated with lower CCOP participation in research-base scientific activities and lower accrual performance.

The development of bonds is the fourth organizing concept. The interaction model characterizes the development of supplier/ customer relationships as a social-exchange process in which the parties gradually demonstrate their trustworthiness to each other and commit themselves to the relationship (Blau, 1964; Hallen, Johanson, and Mohamed, 1987). The need for social exchange is particularly acute when the decision environment is uncertain (Hakansson and Wootz, 1979) and when stability of quality is needed (Hallen, 1980). In addition to trust, CCOPs and research bases may develop technical bonds through joint participation in protocol design, planning bonds, friendship bonds, legal bonds such as formal affiliation agreements, and knowledge-based bonds that allow them to adapt to one another. The need for prompt feedback on patient responses to different treatment regimes creates time-based bonds between the community oncologists who see the patients and the research base investigators who analyze the data. As suggested by social-exchange theory, these bonds result in a "structure of commitments" between the two parties (Hakansson and Ostberg, 1975, p. 115) that assures that they will continue to interact with one another even though they have access to alternative exchange relations (Cook and Emerson, 1984).

Research on CCOP/research-base affiliations helps to clarify the process by which these bonds develop. When a CCOP first affiliates with a research base, the research base may conduct frequent audits of patient data or require that the CCOP register all patients and submit all study forms through a university that will assume responsibility for quality control. As the relationship evolves, the parties tend to become increasingly aware of each other's expectations and capabilities and increasingly trusting of one another. Coordination gradually takes place through planning and friendship bonds rather than through formal agreements and authority systems. These more personal bonds lead to greater cooperation (Hakansson and Johanson, 1988) and a more stable CCOP/research-base relationship.

Hypotheses. Although the interaction model provides a useful framework for analyzing CCOP/research-base reltionships, there is little theoretical understanding of how different types of exchange relate to one another. The following hypotheses suggest how the model can be extended to explain associations between three types of CCOP/research-base exchange (information exchange, protocol exchange, and sociopolitical exchange) and their individual and combined effects on CCOP accrual performance.

Hypothesis 1: Resource dependence will be positively associated with information exchange and protocol exchange. Interorganizational theory suggests that a CCOP will enter into exchange relationships with a research base to gain access to critical resources such as protocols, investigational drugs, and "organizational knowhow" (Pfeffer and Salancik, 1978; Cunningham, 1982a; Hakansson, 1982a; Hagg and Wiedersheim-Paul, 1984). The greater the resource dependence, the more the two parties should engage in direct communications with one another (Van de Ven and Ferry, 1980; Van de Ven and Walker, 1984). These frequent interactions should contribute to intense information flows, as measured by the number of physicians and support staff attending research-base meetings and serving on research-base scientific committees (Morrissey, Hall, and Lindsey, 1982). Information exchange should be particularly intense in the initial stage of the relationship, when the parties are trying to assess each other's resources, capabilities, and expectations (Ford, 1982; Valla, 1986). One would also expect CCOPs with high resource dependence to enroll patients on a greater number of protocols (engage in higher protocol exchange) because of their greater perceived need for new cancer treatments.

Hypothesis 2: Information exchange and protocol exchange will be positively and reciprocally related. By attending research-base meetings and serving on research-base scientific committees,

CCOP physicians obtain information on the objectives, eligibility requirements, and treatment plans of new research protocols. Cunningham and Turnbull (1982) observe that such information exchanges usually precede the exchange of products (or protocols in this study). Face-to-face meetings between CCOP and research-base investigators create opportunities for joint "product" development (Cunningham, 1982b), which should reduce the level of perceived risk in enrolling patients in the protocols and increase the number of different protocols used. High protocol exchange should, in turn, lead to more intensive information exchange because the two parties have to know more about each other's performance and findings (Hakansson, 1982b; Johanson and Wootz, 1986; Hallen, Johanson, and Mohamed, 1987).

Hypothesis 3: Information exchange and protocol exchange will be positively associated with CCOP accrual performance. A number of CCOPs and research bases have noted that community physicians enroll more patients in protocols when they participate in research-base meetings. Meeting attendance and committee service build rich communication channels between CCOP and research-base investigators and increase awareness of new protocols and other members' accrual performance. These direct information exchanges, along with the opportunity to participate in the development of new "products," should make the CCOPs increasingly positive toward and willing to use the protocols (Hakansson, 1987). Findings from the CCOP-I evaluation (Feigl and others, 1987) also suggest that CCOPs engaging in higher protocol exchange (as measured by the number of different protocols used) find it easier to match patients with protocols and, therefore, to increase accrual rates. This multiyear evaluation found a positive relationship between the number of distinct protocols used by a CCOP and its patient accruals.

Hypothesis 4: Information exchange and CCOP accrual performance will be positively associated with subsequent sociopolitical exchange. Within research bases, the ability to influence the decisions or actions of others comes from chairing scientific committees, chairing research protocols, and coauthoring publications. Because CCOPs compete with large universities and with other CCOPs for these opportunities, the appointments reflect both trust and political influence. The interaction model and the social-exchange theory on which it is based suggest that trust is established through personal experiences and the successful execution of product and information exchanges (Ford, 1982; Hakansson, 1982a; Thorelli, 1986). Intensive product exchange in the form of patient accruals increases the probability of social exchange (Hakansson and Wootz, 1979). Information exchange is required both to set up and to maintain the trust (Butler, 1983). Thus, the degree of closeness that a CCOP achieves through information exchange and accrual performance in one period should be a key predictor of the level of sociopolitical exchange in subsequent periods (Cunningham and Homse, 1982).

   Hypothesis 5: High sociopolitical exchange will strengthen the positive association between information exchange, protocol exchange, and CCOP accrual performance. As CCOPs achieve trust and influence within the research base, they should exhibit increased commitment to the relationship. Trust and mutual dependence should accelerate the flow of information (Powell, 1989) and reinforce the perceived need to interact (Hakansson and Wootz, 1979). This trust, commitment, and information sharing should lead to mutual productivity (Spekman, 1988) through increased CCOP accrual performance.

An Organizational-Innovation Perspective on CCOPs

CCOP efficiency in enrolling patients in protocols is a necessary but not a sufficient condition for meeting NCI/DCPC objectives. Long-term viability requires that the CCOPs be institutionalized within their component institutions. To analyze CCOPs as an organizational innovation—a new organizational form invented to solve a particular problem or set of problems (Kimberly, 1987)—researchers can draw on a rich base of innovation theory and research. However, CCOP characteristics such as the rather lengthy period of time required to meet program objectives, their task differentiation (treatment and cancer-control research), and the need for adoption of protocol-based patterns of care by autonomous physicians within the community suggest that we refine our approaches to innovation research in order to understand the major problems confronting these organizational forms. We next present the basic unit of analysis, the problem orientation, and the key concepts of this perspective that need to be considered given the special characteristics of CCOPs.

Basic Unit of Analysis. Although CCOPs are clearly the innovation, they must be analyzed by looking at their component institutions. The hospitals, clinics, and physician group practices that participate in the CCOP are not undifferentiated. Given the interdependence of their activities and the CCOP's reliance on persons, departments, and committees within the components (primary-care physicians and oncologists, medical oncology and radiation-therapy departments, hospital tumor boards), it is important to analyze systematically different units within the components and their differing levels of institutionalization of CCOPs. Both the positive and negative consequences of institutionalization must be considered in this analysis. For example, although institutionalization should assure increased use of protocols within existing facilities, the increased costs to both patient and facilities from meeting protocol requirements may have negative implications. Similarly, the institutionalization of certain protocols that are later found to be ineffective or the inappropriate use of protocols or protocol procedures may adversely affect quality of care. Existing theory—particularly that based on the individual as the unit of analysis—provides little insight into the institutionalization of new organizational forms. The fact that actual and specific manifestations of this process are not well understood is a central problem for programmatic innovations such as CCOPs (Pennings, 1987).

Problem Orientation. Most innovation theories and research have focused on implementation and have used a variance perspective to explain single events (Mohr, 1982). A variance perspective is one in which percent variation in a dependent variable is explained, while a process perspective is one in which evolutionary, chronological, historical change is identified. The time required to meet the programmatic objectives of organizational forms such as CCOPs directs attention to the innovation process and requires new analytical approaches that resemble what Mohr (1982) calls process theories. Emphasis needs to be placed on a series of events as proximate causes in the innovation process in addition to adopter characteristics and attributes of the innovation itself. The innovation process and the manner in which it unfolds over time may be the ultimate determinant of subsequent events.

Another issue that requires attention is the character of the innovation itself. CCOPs, as organizational innovations, are expected to conduct two distinct kinds of activities—treatment research and cancer-control research. The first activity (treating patients) is quite compatible with traditional health care services, while the second (promoting population-based behavior change) requires significant departures from accepted and ongoing medical activities. The distinct attributes of each type of activity and their differing effects on CCOP institutionalization challenge the view that organizational innovations have just one set of attributes and help to explain why previous innovation studies have produced conflicting findings.

Key Concepts. The analysis of CCOP institutionalization requires new approaches to innovation theory that are based on three basic concepts. The first is the concept of stages. The designation of CCOP activities as an organizational innovation focuses attention on the institutionalization process over time rather than as a single event. Although investigators in the organizational-innovation tradition do not agree on the exact number of stages in the innovation process or their characteristics, they generally agree that the process involves multiple decisions and actions over a period of time. Most models begin with an awareness or knowledge stage, continue with an adoption or decision stage, which includes some aspects of implementation, and conclude with an institutionalization stage, which focuses on the integration of the innovation into ongoing organizational activities (Zaltman, Duncan, and Holbek, 1973; Scheirer, 1983; Kaluzny and Hernandez, 1988; Goodman and Steckler, 1989). Because the CCOP organizational form requires the participation of autonomous physicians in an interorganizational setting, it must be accepted not only by the component institutions but also by individual physicians who will refer patients to specific treatment and cancer-control protocols. Thus, there is a second decision point at which the CCOP, as an organizational innovation, must be accepted.

The second concept is that of types of change. Innovation is not an undifferentiated phenomenon. Innovative programs that are consistent with ongoing objectives of the organization tend to be implemented, while innovations that affect or change ongoing objectives encounter resistance and difficulty (Kaluzny and Veney, 1977; Nathanson and Morlock, 1980; Greer, 1988). In the case of CCOP, although both the treatment and cancer-control research activities are part of the expected behavior in this innovative program, the treatment activities are far more consistent with ongoing service-delivery activities in community hospitals and physician practices than are the cancer-control activities. Cancer-control research requires significantly different organizational goals and operating procedures to implement and institutionalize within component organizations.

A third concept is that of secondary effects. Organizational innovation may not affect the entire organization. Because innovation typically affects only some units within a larger organizational context, recognition of the contingent nature of the implementation decision is important (Rogers, 1983). For example, the CCOP involves autonomous physicians and hospital administrators, each of whom can influence how and when the innovation is implemented by referring patients or allocating resources. This contingent aspect draws attention to the fact that CCOP component institutions are more than simply rational structures pursuing a priori goals; they are political systems composed of coalitions and interest groups, each pursuing its own agenda (Fennell and Warnecke, 1988). The relative success of CCOP institutionalization in component institutions depends, to a great extent, on its compatibility with these different groups' goals and priorities. Likewise, the prospects for CCOP institutionalization in the larger community depend on CCOP compatibility with area physicians' goals and practice patterns.

Hypotheses. Although innovation research and theory provide a useful analytical framework, the characteristics of CCOPs suggest several areas for theoretical development and testing. These areas are summarized in the following hypotheses:

Hypothesis 6: The degree of CCOP institutionalization will be influenced by prior stages of the innovation process, and the manner in which the program is implemented will affect program outcomes. Innovation is a nonrecursive process. Because various stages feed into each other, prior stages are important determinants of subsequent stages of innovation, including the ultimate impact. Institutionalization is most likely to occur when significant actors within organizations recognize a problem and identify a particular innovation as a resolution to that problem. In the case of CCOPs, component recognition that there is a problem with the quality of care being provided within the community is a critical precursor to institutionalization.

For CCOPs, institutionalization is not the end result but an interim event leading to changes in physician practice patterns. With these changes as the ultimate outcome, the time element becomes important, suggesting that those factors that directly affect the duration of any particular stage in the overall innovation process will be most critical. One such factor is how the CCOP is implemented. Although we will be testing this hypothesis with data from the CCOP-II evaluation, preliminary site-visit findings provide tentative support. For example, CCOPs that had relationships with research bases prior to the establishment of the program that developed explicit procedures for protocol selection and ranking during the initial implementation phase seem to be experiencing the fewest problems in meeting accrual requirements and winning physician and component acceptance.

Hypothesis 7: Component organizations that have both well-established cancer-control activities and highly specialized, formalized, and centralized structures will quickly institutionalize the CCOP. Viewing CCOPs as organizational innovations requires differentiation of the types of activities CCOPs are expected to perform. When CCOP activities involve protocol-based treatment, the innovation represents an expansion of the usual activity for hospital units. However, when clinical activities are integrated with cancer-control research, in such areas as early detection, prevention, and behavioral change, they require resource and personnel commitments not directly under the control of the medical specialists to whom the award is made. Persuading surgeons and other primary-care physicians to participate in cancer-control research requires significant organizational commitment at several levels of the hierarchy. Moreover, it is important to consider the role of organizational structure in the institutionalization process. Specialization, formalization, and centralization within an organization are frequently cited as barriers to implementation; yet these same features can also support the orderly introduction of innovations (Scott, 1990). When an innovation is consistent with the established goals of the organization and an appropriate structure is in place, the innovation is likely to be quickly implemented.

Hypothesis 8: The implementation of the CCOP will have different effects on the various functional areas of component organizations, and where there is mutual adaptation institutionalization will be maximized. The diversity of interests in organizations affects the extent to which innovations are implemented by various functional areas. The degree of consistency between different groups' agendas and their expectations of CCOPs determines the extent to which the CCOP is integrated into component organizations. A CCOP's inclusion of personnel from disciplines such as epidemiology and the psychosocial sciences in cancer-control research may threaten some medical specialties within component hospitals. Moreover, the need to involve primary-care physicians in cancer-control research further complicates the process and may produce conflict between health professionals over roles and areas of authority.

When there is mutual adaptation, in which both the CCOP and its component organizations make accommodations, institutionalization will be enhanced. As described by one hospital administrator in a multicomponent CCOP: "We are a team, and we work as a group community program. It would be perceived as offensive to any of us if one hospital started saying, 'We're the only CCOP hospital.' By virtue of that, we have talked about it and said, 'Okay, when we release something to the newspapers, everyone will release it at the same time.' When we do some sort of article [on the CCOP], it is approved through all the channels. Everybody sees it; everybody has access to it. It's not written down that this is what you have to do and these are the people who have to check on it, but I think, from a political standpoint, you have to be sensitive to that."

Integrating Interaction and Innovation Perspectives

This analysis of CCOP/research-base relations and the institutionalization of CCOPs in component organizations highlights certain deficiencies in the interaction and innovation perspectives along with the need to push for their integration. Despite distinctive emphases, the two theoretical models are complementary. They have a common origin in social-learning theory, and they both call attention to developmental stages, resource dependencies, mutual adaptation, and the need for time-dependent, process analyses. Because the core organizing processes that each model focuses on (innovation and adaptation) are causally interrelated in most social organizational settings, a synthesis of the two perspectives is possible on both conceptual and empirical grounds.

We have presented the (internal) functioning of CCOPs and their (external) relations with research bases as if the two processes were discrete activities. In fact, both occur simultaneously, and events and processes from one arena can have profound implications for outcomes in the other. For example, unless CCOP physicians develop mechanisms within their host institutions for ensuring a steady flow of patient enrollments in protocols and high-quality protocol data (the adoption and institutionalization phases of innovation theory), the long-term relationships and structure of commitments between CCOPs and their research bases (as envisioned by the interaction model) will have little opportunity to emerge and mature. Similarly, if research bases are slow in developing cancer-control research protocols or if they design protocols that require a special mix of local organizations or professionals (for example, oncologists and hospitals as well as health maintenance organizations, primary-care physicians, epidemiologists, and community health educators), then the pace and complexity of the adoption and institutionalization processes will be mitigated for some CCOPs and intensified for others.

Once the reciprocal influence between CCOP institutionalization and research-base relationships is recognized, we can begin to identify research questions that extend, refine, and integrate the two theoretical models. For example, is there something about the implementation of these particular organizational forms that predetermines CCOP/research-base exchange patterns or the level of CCOP institutionalization? Similarly, is a particular CCOP/research-base exchange pattern associated with different levels of institutionalization? One plausible hypothesis is that CCOPs where cancer-treatment research is well integrated into component organizations will experience the most difficulty in adopting and institutionalizing the new cancer-control research protocols. Another is that sociopolitical exchanges involving close collaboration between CCOP and research-base investigators (in protocol design, joint publications, committee work) promote high levels of commitment to cancer research and easy institutionalization of the CCOP in its component institutions.

The ultimate utility of these new insights into organizational theory can be seen in their implications for future health-services research and the management of new organizational forms. Some of the promise in each domain is highlighted in the concluding sections of this chapter.

Research Implications. To this point, we have focused on only two of the social relationships in which CCOPs are embedded: the interorganizational relationship between CCOPs and their research bases and the intraorganizational relationships between CCOP physicians and their component institutions (medical practices and community hospitals). Several other sets and levels of relationships involving CCOPs can be usefully analyzed from innovation, interaction, or hybrid perspectives.

CCOP innovation can be viewed as an interorganizational phenomenon rather than as a process occurring within single organizations (Knoke and Kuklinski, 1982). Here, the basic unit of analysis shifts from the individual organization to the collectivity of organizations. Attention focuses on the local CCOP as the adopted or innovative unit and the ways in which the composition and structure of the components (medical practices and hospitals) influence the probability, pace, and outcomes of the innovation-institutionalization process. Such an analysis provides an opportunity to extend existing theory into the realm of interorganizational innovation, an area that has not received much attention to date. Whether existing propositions from innovation and interaction theories can be extrapolated to the interorganizational level, and whether new variables and relationships are required to account for variations in network adoption behaviors would be among the central analytical questions guiding empirical work.

A network focus on CCOPs raises questions about the extent to which local CCOPs are physician-based or organization-based systems. A major theme that emerged from our early fieldwork is that CCOPs are physician-dominated organizations that are constrained by the private practice of medicine. Most participants are full-time physicians and part-time researchers. Although trained in clinical-trials methods and committed to research-based medicine, CCOP investigators are practicing physicians faced with the economic exigencies of maintaining private practices and minimizing competition for patients and fees. These economic considerations exert strong influences on which local physicians and hospitals participate in the CCOP, and they may well influence physician receptivity to population-based versus patient-based cancer-control research.

At the same time, CCOP component hospitals are often competitors in the marketplace. We were struck by the fact that relatively few interhospital relationships exist outside of the CCOP, and that CCOPs have not stimulated new collaborations among the component institutions. In most instances, hospitals are drawn into the CCOPs through their affiliated physicians; several administrators acknowledged that if their oncologists were not committed to the CCOP the hospitals would have little or no incentive for investing scarce resources in joint research. At the same time, most hospital administrators recognize that the CCOP is good for marketing purposes and that it helps to project the image that state-of-the-art cancer care is available at local community hospitals. Here we have an instance of a "parallel organization" (Shortell, 1985) that physicians and hospital administrators create to accomplish goals that cannot be accommodated within the typical general hospital structure.

These considerations suggest that CCOPs can be arrayed along a continuum ranging from relatively informal physician collaborations to formal arrangements in which CCOP performance rests on interorganizational as well as interphysician relationships. In the context of the issues discussed in this chapter, the interesting questions have to do with the ways in which innovation and interaction processes vary for CCOPs at different points along this continuum. Do the CCOPs that are organized as formal interorganizational structures have a higher rate of adoption for cancer-control protocols than those with informal structures? Are informal systems more effective in linking community oncologists and primary-care physicians so that cancer-control practices are more quickly diffused to the large physician community?

Opportunities for research are also available at another level. In addition to CCOPs and research bases, the NCI constitutes a third arm of the cancer-research program. NCI develops the national research agenda, reviews and approves cancer-treatment and cancer-control protocols, funds CCOPs and research bases, and monitors progress toward its goals. The relationships and interdependencies among the three entities influence the organizational performance of each member as well as the overall success of the national cancer-research program. For research purposes, each paired relationship can be analyzed as a separate phenomenon. In this chapter, we have devoted attention exclusively to the CCOP/research-base relationship, but the innovation and interaction perspectives are equally applicable to CCOP/NCI and research-base/NCI relationships. Each relationship has its own developmental stages, resource dependencies, mutual adaptations, and institutionalization issues. Following the logic we applied to the local CCOPs, it is a short step conceptually to aggregate these triadic relationships to the level of a national interorganizational network for cancer-control and cancer-treatment research. As we move through these increasingly inclusive relational levels, emergent processes or phenomena at each higher level require new explanatory frameworks or modifications of existing theory.

Management Implications. Thus far we have addressed the theoretical and research insights arising from our early fieldwork on the CCOP. Our mandate as evaluators is to identify the characteristics of successful CCOPs and the factors that NCI program managers can manipulate to enhance the overall performance of the local programs. Our analyses suggest that the CCOP is a complex, multifaceted, and multitiered interorganizational system that encompasses a number of stakeholders who have partially overlapping and partially independent agendas. Consequently, the management of this enterprise and the effort to move it forward toward unified goals and performance targets are formidable and uncertain tasks.

Some of the oppositional forces and obstacles to achieving these management goals can be highlighted by looking at the range of stakeholders that must be attended to in this process. At the local level, we have community oncologists, who are part of a new cadre of well-trained and outcome-oriented physician-researchers who must balance the political economy of private practice with the organizational thrust to link physicians and hospitals in a joint cancer-research program. Research bases are large, geographically dispersed, and fluid organizational structures that combine aspects of "invisible colleges," franchises, and university consortia. Here, the predominant focus is on the science of oncology and the design of research protocols that can advance the frontiers of knowledge. The tension within research bases revolves around the competition among investigators for scientific breakthroughs and the necessity to mount collaborative efforts to assemble the large-sample data bases needed to evaluate the efficacy and effectiveness of new agents, clinical procedures, and practices. In addition, for research scientists, cancer-control research may not be a top-priority effort given the promise of other basic or treatment-oriented studies. The NCI, in turn, is charged with multiple and at times conflicting mandates: fostering science, diffusing new knowledge to practicing physicians, and managing a national research and education program. Each stakeholder group aligns with professional and political interest groups to further common goals and priority concerns and looks to staff units within the NCI to champion its interests in the resource-allocation and agenda-setting processes. The challenge for NCI program managers is to find ways to mobilize the research community behind its national agenda while identifying incentives that will encourage the adoption of best-practice procedures by community physicians. Herding cats may well be an easier task!

In conclusion, the CCOP affords an opportunity to describe and analyze a variety of new organizational forms that are coming to dominate the landscape of health care and health-services research. In many ways, these entities and their interrelationships afford opportunities to test, refine, and extend current organization theory and to develop new knowledge for the management of these multicomponent and multifaceted enterprises. Our ongoing research will address many of the issues raised in this chapter, and the results of this work will, we hope, point to new avenues for the development of organization theory.

References

Axelsson, B. "Supplier Management and Technological Development." In H. Hakansson (ed.), *Industrial Technological Development: A Network Approach*. London: Croom Helm, 1987.

Blau, P. M. *Exchange and Power in Social Life*. New York: Wiley, 1964.

Butler, R. "A Transactional Approach to Organizing Efficiency: Perspectives from Markets, Hierarchies, and Collectives." *Administration and Society*, 1983, *15*, 323–362.

Cook, K. S. "Emerson's Contributions to Social Exchange Theory." In K. S. Cook (ed.), *Social Exchange Theory*. Beverly Hills, Calif.: Sage, 1987.

Cook, K. S., and Emerson, R. M. "Exchange Networks and the Analysis of Complex Organizations." In S. B. Bacharach and E. J. Lawler (eds.), *Research in the Sociology of Organizations*. Vol. 3. Greenwich, Conn.: JAI, 1984.

Cunningham, M. T. "An Interaction Approach to Purchasing Strategy." In H. Hakansson (ed.), *International Marketing and Purchasing of Industrial Goods: An Interaction Approach*. New York: Wiley, 1982a.

Cunningham, M. T. "Barriers to Organizational Interaction." In H. Hakansson (ed.), *International Marketing and Purchasing of Industrial Goods: An Interaction Approach*. New York: Wiley, 1982b.

Cunningham, M. T., and Homse, E. "An Interaction Approach to Marketing Strategy." In H. Hakansson (ed.), *International Marketing and Purchasing of Industrial Goods: An Interaction Approach.* New York: Wiley, 1982.

Cunningham, M. T., and Turnbull, P. W. "Interorganizational Personal Contact Patterns." In H. Hakansson (ed.), *International Marketing and Purchasing of Industrial Goods: An Interaction Approach.* New York: Wiley, 1982.

Feigl, P., and others. *Community Cancer Care Evaluation (CCCE), Final Report.* Vol. 5: *Integrated Analysis.* National Cancer Institute Contract N01-CN-35009. Seattle: Statistical Analysis and Quality Control Center, Fred Hutchinson Cancer Research Center, 1987.

Fennell, M., and Warnecke, R. *The Diffusion of Medical Innovation: An Applied Network Analysis.* New York: Plenum, 1988.

Ford, D. "The Development of Buyer-Seller Relationships in Industrial Markets." In H. Hakansson (ed.), *International Marketing and Purchasing of Industrial Goods: An Interaction Approach.* New York: Wiley, 1982.

Goodman, R. M., and Steckler, A. "A Framework for Assessing Program Institutionalization." *Knowledge in Society,* 1989, *2* (1), 52–66.

Greer, A. L. "The State of the Art Versus the State of the Science." *International Journal of Technology Assessment in Health Care,* 1988, *4,* 5–26.

Hagg, I., and Wiedersheim-Paul, F. "Introduction." In I. Hagg and F. Wiedersheim-Paul (eds.), *Between Market and Hierarchy.* Uppsala, Sweden: Uppsala University, 1984.

Hakansson, H. "An Interaction Approach." In H. Hakansson (ed.), *International Marketing and Purchasing of Industrial Goods: An Interaction Approach.* New York: Wiley, 1982a.

Hakansson, H. "Interaction Themes: The Company Cases and the Interaction Model—An Overview." In H. Hakansson (ed.), *International Marketing and Purchasing of Industrial Goods: An Interaction Approach.* New York: Wiley, 1982b.

———. "Technological Innovation Through Interaction." In H. Hakansson (ed.), *Industrial Technological Development: A Network Approach.* London: Croom Helm, 1987.

Hakansson, H., and Johanson, J. "Formal and Informal Cooperation Strategies in International Industrial Networks." In F. Contractor and P. Lorange (eds.), *Cooperative Strategies in International Business.* Lexington, Mass.: Lexington Books, 1988.

Hakansson, H., and Ostberg, C. "Industrial Marketing: An Organizational Problem?" *Industrial Marketing Management,* 1975, *4,* 113–123.

Hakansson, H., and Wootz, B. "A Framework of Industrial Buying and Selling." *Industrial Marketing Management,* 1979, *8,* 28–39.

Hallen, L. "Stability and Change in Supplier Relationships." In L. Engwall and J. Johanson (eds.), *Some Aspects of Control in International Business.* Uppsala, Sweden: Almqvist and Wiksell, 1980.

Hallen, L., Johanson, J., and Mohamed, N. S. "Relationship Strength and Stability in International and Domestic Industrial Marketing." *Industrial Marketing and Purchasing,* 1987, *2,* 22–37.

Hallen, L., and Wiedersheim-Paul, F. "The Evolution of Psychic Distance in International Business Relationships." In I. Hagg and F. Wiedersheim-Paul (eds.), *Between Market and Hierarchy.* Uppsala, Sweden: Uppsala University, 1984.

Hannan, M. T., and Freeman, J. "Structural Inertia and Organizational Change." *American Sociological Review,* 1984, *49,* 149–164.

Johanson, J. "Business Relationships and Industrial Networks: Observations in International Business Research." In *Perspectives on the Economics of Organization, Crafoord Lectures 1.* Lund, Sweden: Lund University Press, 1988.

Johanson, J., and Mattsson, L. "Interorganizational Relations in Industrial Systems: A Network Approach Compared with the Transaction-Cost Approach." *International Studies of Management and Organization,* 1987, *27,* 34–48.

Johanson, J., and Wootz, B. "The German Approach to Europe." In P. Turnbull and J. P. Valla (eds.), *Strategies for International Industrial Marketing: The Management of Customer Relationships in European Industrial Markets.* London: Croom Helm, 1986.

Kaluzny, A. D., and Hernandez, S. R. "Organizational Change and Innovation." In S. Shortell and A. Kaluzny (eds.), *Health Care Management*, (2nd ed.). New York: Wiley, 1988.

Kaluzny, A. D. and Veney, J. "Types of Change and Hospital Planning Strategies." *American Journal of Health Planning*, 1977, *1*, 13–19.

Kaluzny, A. D., and others. "Evaluating Organizational Design to Assure Technology Transfer: The Case of the Community Clinical Oncology Program." *Journal of the National Cancer Institute*, 1989, *81*, 1717–1725.

Kimberly, J. R. "Organizational and Contextual Influences on the Diffusion of Technology Innovation." In J. Pennings and A. Buitendam (eds.), *New Technology as Organizational Innovation*. Cambridge, Mass.: Ballinger, 1987.

Kimberly, J. R., Miles, R., and associates. *The Organizational Life Cycle*. San Francisco: Jossey-Bass, 1980.

Knoke, D., and Kuklinski, J. *Network Analysis*. Beverly Hills, Calif.: Sage, 1982.

Laage-Hellman, J. "Process Innovation Through Technical Cooperation." In H. Hakansson (ed.), *Industrial Technological Development: A Network Approach*. London: Croom Helm, 1987.

Mohr, L. T. *Explaining Organizational Behavior*. San Francisco: Jossey-Bass, 1982.

Morrissey, J. P., Hall, R. H., and Lindsey, M. L. *Interorganizational Relations: A Sourcebook of Measures for Mental Health Programs*. Department of Health and Human Services Publication (ADM) 82-1187. Washington, D.C.: U.S. Government Printing Office, 1982.

Nathanson, C., and Morlock, L. "Control Structures, Values, and Innovation." *Journal of Health and Social Behavior*, 1980, *21* (4), 315–333.

Pennings, J. M. "On the Nature of New Technology as Organizational Innovation." In J. Pennings and A. Buitendam (eds.), *New Technology as Organizational Innovation*. Cambridge, Mass.: Ballinger, 1987.

Pfeffer, J., and Salancik, G. R. *The External Control of Organizations: A Resource Dependence Perspective*. New York: Harper & Row, 1978.

Powell, W. W. "Neither Market nor Hierarchy: Network Forms of Organization." In B. M. Staw and L. L. Cummings (eds.), *Research in Organizational Behavior.* Vol. 12. Greenwich, Conn.: JAI, 1989.

Rogers, E. M. *Diffusion of Innovations.* (3rd ed.) New York: Free Press, 1983.

Scheirer, M. A. "Approaches to the Study of Implementation." *IEEE Transactions in Engineering Management,* 1983, *30,* 76–82.

Scott, W. R. "Innovation in Medical Care Organizations: A Synthetic Review." *Medical Care Review,* forthcoming, 1990.

Shortell, S. M. "The Medical Staff of the Future: Replanting the Garden." *Frontiers of Health Services Management,* 1985, *1,* 3–48.

Spekman, R. E. "Strategic Supplier Selection: Understanding Long-Term Buyer Relationships." *Business Horizons,* 1988, *31,* 75–81.

Thorelli, H. B. "Networks: Between Markets and Hierarchies." *Strategic Management Journal,* 1986, *7,* 37–51.

University of North Carolina, Health Services Research Center. *Community Clinical Oncology Program Key Informant Study.* Chapel Hill: Health Services Research Center, University of North Carolina, 1988.

Valla, J. P. "The French Approach to Europe." In P. Turnbull and J. P. Valla (eds.), *Strategies for International Industrial Marketing: The Management of Customer Relationships in European Industrial Markets.* London: Croom Helm, 1986.

Van de Ven, A., and Ferry, D. *Measuring and Assessing Organizations.* New York: Wiley, 1980.

Van de Ven, A., and Walker, G. "The Dynamics of Interorganizational Coordination." *Administrative Science Quarterly,* 1984, *29,* 598–621.

Weick, K. E. *The Social Psychology of Organizing.* New York: Random House, 1979.

Wilson, D., and Mummalaneni, V. "Bonding and Commitment in Buyer-Seller Relationships: A Preliminary Conceptualization." *Industrial Marketing and Purchasing,* 1986, *1,* 44–58.

Zaltman, G., Duncan, R., and Holbek, J. *Innovations and Organizations.* New York: Wiley, 1973.

5

Structure and Strategy in Hospital-Physician Relationships

James W. Begun
Roice D. Luke
Dennis D. Pointer

Organizations have a variety of configurations and ways of functioning, illustrated best perhaps by the eight metaphors or images forwarded by Morgan (1986) (among them, machines, organisms, political systems). Characterizing an organization becomes increasingly complex as interactions with other organizations are brought into the description. For instance, where one organization begins and another ends is difficult to ascertain. Yet interactions with other organizations are a vital part of the reality of any organization, given its need to secure resources and distribute products or services. Hospitals, in particular, interact with a wide variety of organizations to assure their own viability and to facilitate the proper functioning of a complex patient-care system.

In contrast to most other organizations, hospitals also interact extensively with a powerful and distinct occupational group—physicians. For this reason, the hospital/physician relationship has been a subject of great interest for many years. Although relationships with physicians have long been among the most important interdependencies faced by hospitals, only recently have these relationships assumed major strategic importance in the health care marketplace. Today the hospital/physician relationship is, arguably, the most important organizational feature of hospitals because of multiple patient-care and financial interdependencies and the

116

impact physicians have on efficiency and effectiveness. The design and management of hospital/physician relationships have become major determinants of competitive success for many hospitals and for physicians. New forms of hospital/physician relationships are emerging, thereby prompting the need for new ways to conceptualize them.

How can the evolving patterns of relationships between hospitals and physicians best be characterized? In this chapter we develop a typology of interorganizational forms that includes four types of organization/professional relationships. The classification scheme is based on the structural and strategic dimensions of these relationships. After using the typology to examine trends in hospital/physician relationships, we explore distinctive management and research issues arising from application of the typology.

We hope to contribute to research and management in the following ways. First, our typology adds to, and strengthens, the growing conceptual literature in organization theory that focuses on nonbureaucratic interorganizational links such as strategic alliances, quasi-firms, and networks. In particular, the typology directly incorporates the dimension of strategic purpose into the classification of organizational forms. Health care examples illuminate and extend this literature because the health care sector is in the forefront of developing new forms of loosely coupled but strategic interorganizational relationships (Luke, Begun, and Pointer, 1989).

Second, the discussion contributes to the literature on the role of professionals in organizations. We argue that the hospital/physician relationship, when viewed within a radically changing external environment, must be reassessed. Given the changing environment and evolving hospital/physician structures that increase coordination and control yet preserve the essential autonomy of physicians, it becomes useful to conceive of physicians as other than (potential or actual) labor inputs. To the extent that any workers are strategically important to an organization and have a high degree of occupational autonomy, they must be viewed in an interorganizational framework. Conceptualizing autonomous professionals as strategic organizational units may lessen the utility of the concept of professional in organization theory.

Finally, effective management of organization/professional relationships is more strategically significant in health care today than ever before, but the conceptual tools available to handle these relationships are weak. This weakness may pertain because many of the current hospital/physician links are new and because practice is changing faster than theory. Health care administrators need typologies of hospital/physician (or organization/professional) relationships in order to identify and understand the alternative forms these relationships might take, the relative assets and liabilities of each alternative form, and the management responses that might be appropriate in particular situations. Managers in other industries also can draw on and learn from health care organizational innovations in structuring and managing relationships with autonomous professionals.

Conceptualizing Hospital/Physician Relationships

In this section, we review approaches to understanding and managing diverse relationships between organizations and professionals. The term *professional* is a "historically and nationally specific 'folk concept'" (Freidson, 1986). In this chapter we mean professionals to include those individuals whose work is highly specialized, is based on extensive training, and is relatively immune from outside control during the production process. Immunity from outside control (professional autonomy) can derive from task characteristics or from the political and social power of the profession. In either case, organizational managers must deal with claims of professional autonomy by the worker.

In general, professionals' autonomy from organizational control has been viewed along a continuum, ranging from high autonomy, in the case of such professions as medicine, to low autonomy, in the case of such professions as engineering. Scott's (1982; 1987, pp. 236–238) three-category scheme of organization/professional relationships is illustrative. Autonomous professional control exists when the organization delegates a substantial degree of control to the professional group. Heteronomous relationships are defined by administrative control of the professional group in a hierarchy, with relatively little autonomy granted to professionals.

Conjoint relationships reflect a pluralist rather than a hierarchical structure, with multiple centers of power. Contemporary hospital/medical staff relationships are conjoint (Griffith, 1987).

Mintzberg's (1979, 1983) popular structural typology of organizations includes one type in which professionals are present in large numbers, the professional bureaucracy. In it, hierarchical control does not extend down into the professionalized production core. Instead, professional socialization and autonomy create a self-regulatory structure. Interdependent administrative hierarchies may emerge, one democratic and bottom-up for the professionals, and another machine bureaucratic and top-down for support staff. Professional bureaucracies may exist in universities, general hospitals, school systems, public accounting firms, social-work agencies, and craft production firms (Mintzberg, 1983, p. 189).

Much of the management literature deals with controlling and integrating professionals in organizational settings. A large literature describes management approaches to resolving the "misfit" between professional work and bureaucratic structure (for example, Benveniste, 1987; Katz, 1988; Mills, Hall, Leidecker, and Margulies, 1983; Raelin, 1986; Sheldon, 1986). Such approaches include less reliance on formal controls and more reliance on intrinsic motivation, trust, and professional and ethical controls; increased emphasis on conflict resolution, team building, and consensus building; decentralization; job enrichment; and the placement of professionals in key administrative positions (board member, chief executive officer) or in organization/professional liaison positions (the medical director in a hospital). The general goal of these approaches is to incorporate the professional directly into the structure and functioning of the organization. Virtually all these tactics have been recommended for the cementing of hospital/physician relationships (for example, Herbert-Carter, 1988).

Overall, these past perspectives on organization/professional relationships have been useful in characterizing the degree to which organizations are able to incorporate professionals as labor inputs. Past conceptualizations of the hospital/physician relationship, similarly, view physicians primarily as labor in the hospital's production process. These conceptualizations include Scott's typology, already discussed. A dual line of authority is said to exist in the hospital, with management exerting control over support functions and physicians controlling clinical functions (Harris, 1977; Smith, 1955). The triad model of hospital governance, which identifies the medical staff and administration as separate corners of a triangle, both reporting to the governing board at the apex of the triangle, also depicts the attempt to incorporate physicians as labor into the hospital organization (for example, Rakich, Longest, and Darr, 1985, pp. 177–180).

More recent perspectives on hospital/physician relationships include two that are based largely on the degree of management control exerted by the hospital over the physicians. Shortell's (1985) categories place the medical staff as an organization solely within the hospital, both within and separate, or solely separate. In the Glandon and Morrisey (1986) undimensional scheme, which places physicians on a continuum from autonomous to supervised hospital, control over physicians is strongest when the physicians are employed. Hospital control is weakest when physicians are not employed and only share a common interest with the hospital, but control is enhanced by limiting access to the hospital to selected physicians (for example, the most cost-effective ones) and by creating a formal hospital/physician organization.

Several important factors distinguish hospital/physician relationships from other organization/professional relationships and argue for a broad conceptualization of hospital/physician interaction. The complex and critical nature of physicians' work, the high level of professionalism and power achieved by physicians, the often unassailable autonomy granted to them, and their unmatched ability to shift their allegiance from one affiliated organization to another have forged for physicians a far different relationship with hospitals than that experienced by other health care workers, including many that fall within the professional category. The contrast between physicians and other professionals who work outside of health care may be the same. Lawyers, research scientists, and engineers, for instance, do not have the same ability to withdraw from their affiliated organizations that physicians possess.

The unusually powerful position of physicians relative to hospitals has been widely recognized. For instance, Pauly and Redisch (1973, p. 88), in their classic description of the hospital as a physicians' cooperative, treat physicians essentially as outsiders who are so autonomous that they actually enjoy *"de facto* control of the hospital."* Scott (1982, p. 216) declares that the "separation of professional and administrative jurisdictions is more clearly exemplified by U.S. hospitals than any other type of organization." Quite telling is the fact that many organizational charts of hospitals do not even include physicians on them, or they indicate a dotted-line relationship between the medical staff as a group and the chief executive officer or governing board.

As the external environment of hospitals and other health care organizations becomes increasingly threatening and uncertain, it is reasonable to expect that the organizations will attempt to restructure their relationships with physicians to increase control (Burchell, White, Smith, and Piland, 1988). Such restructuring can be expected to take one of two forms: either a more market-oriented or a more bureaucratic set of interrelationships—the classic choice between markets and hierarchies to mediate exchanges (Williamson, 1975).

The shift toward a more bureaucratic form would draw physicians into a traditional organization/employee relationship with hospitals. To use Scott's terminology, the relationships would become more heteronomous if they currently are conjoint, or more conjoint if they currently are autonomous, and a consequence would be some erosion in physician autonomy. The bureaucratization of many hospital/physician relationships is a widely acknowledged trend today. For instance, Alexander, Morrisey, and Shortell (1986, p. 233) state that "while most physicians will remain nonemployees, . . . they are fast becoming . . . organizational members" through increased integration into hospital structures.

Less commonly appreciated, however, is the fact that physicians can become organizational members in a strategic sense through looser, rather than tighter, coupling with hospitals. The growth of loosely coupled, strategically important hospital/physician organizations, reviewed later in this chapter, illustrates that shared strategic goals can be met without the tight coupling inherent in bureaucratic organizations. A move toward more market-oriented relationships causes the separate physician structure implicit in the conjoint organization to, in effect, become more external. In other words, the parallel physician and hospital structures implicit in the conjoint organization are increasingly coordinated through contractual and other market arrangements rather than by intraorganizational agreement. Physicians (either individually or collectively) thus begin to function more as if they were independent, potentially competitive business firms than as professional employees or staff of hospitals. These increasingly externalized units have to assume a strategic orientation to hospitals, other organizations, and the environment generally. They are driven by their own as well as collective (joint hospital and physician) strategic purposes, compete alongside other firms in the marketplace, and interact with other organizations, as necessary, to achieve individual or collective strategic purposes or both.

Past conceptualizations of organization/professional relationships were developed and applied to physicians and other professionals in an era in which the external environment was relatively passive. But with a rapidly changing environment, the informal links between the organization and its professionals need to be strengthened through the addition of either increasingly formal bureaucratic structures or traditional market mechanisms.

All these developments argue for treating hospital/physician relationships as a class of organization/organization, rather than organization/professional, relationships. For this reason, we turn to conceptualizations of relationships between organizations that share strategic interdependencies.

A General Typology of Organization/Professional Relationships

Classifications of interorganizational forms, let alone of organization/professional relationships, generally have not fully addressed the strategic dimension of most interorganizational relationships. Recent work, however, notes the strategic importance of interorganizational collectives and identifies new hybrid interorganizational relationships, most often classified as "strategic alliances" or "strategic networks" (Astley and Fombrun, 1983; Astley, 1984; Borys and Jemison, 1989; Jarillo, 1988, Kanter, 1989; Miles and Snow, 1986; Powell, 1987; Thorelli, 1986). For example, Miles and Snow (1986, p. 62) describe a new organizational form, the dynamic network, that is "a unique combination of *strategy*, structure and management processes" [emphasis added]. Borys and Jemison (1989) define hybrids as organizational arrangements that use resources or governance structures or both from more than one existing organization. They argue that hybrids can be distinguished by their breadth of purpose, with the following types arrayed from narrowest to broadest: mergers and acquisitions, joint ventures, license agreements, and supplier arrangements. Jarillo (1988) describes strategic networks as nonhierarchical alternatives to market relationships for organizing economic activity. Partners interested in long-term, relatively unstructured relationships and who want to remain as independent organizations may find it economically efficient to form strategic networks.

The growing recognition of the importance of strategy in the classification of alternative forms of interorganizational relationships has yet to be reflected in applications to organization/professional or, more specifically, to hospital/physician relationships. To correct for this oversight, we suggest that organization/professional relationships can be conceptualized employing two dimensions: structure and strategy. In previous work (Luke, Begun, and Pointer, 1989; Pointer, Begun, and Luke, 1988), we treated interorganizational relationships as varying along a structural dimension, measured by a continuum of tight to loose coupling. In a broad sense, the degree of coupling is analogous to the "tensile strength" or "stickiness of the glue" binding the entities (Weick, 1976). In a tightly coupled relationship, the separate boundaries of the joined parties are transcended by a new organizational boundary. In a loosely coupled relationship, joined parties maintain their separate boundaries even while they are responsive to each other. The systems theorists' descriptions of dependence between systems is useful: Two systems are coupled if they share common variables or if variables in one system change in ways related to the alteration of any variable in the second system (Glassman, 1973; Miller, 1978). For example, professionals tightly coupled with their organization might share physical space and support facilities (common variables), and changes in the client base of the organization might affect the client base of the professionals (correlated alteration of variables). Loosely coupled professionals would share fewer common variables with the organization than tightly coupled professionals, and the actions of each party would be more independent. Although the concept of coupling obviously combines many different aspects of organization/professional relationships, we focus on its structural manifestations.

In addition to the structural dimensions, interorganizational relationships serve varying degrees of strategic purpose, as defined by two dimensions: the permanence and the importance of the arrangement. Intended permanence and perceived high importance are two necessary conditions for the purpose of a relationship to be strategic. The notion of strategic purpose is consistent with Mintzberg's (1987) use of the term *intended strategy,* as distinguished from *emergent strategy* or *realized strategy.* A relationship is strategic if it is intended or perceived to be so, even if it does not actually emerge as a realized strategic relationship. Furthermore, it cannot truly be considered strategic a priori if it is not intended to be so. Once realized, it should be considered a strategic relationship in fact.

Both intended permanence and perceived importance of a relationship may be difficult to assess. Strategic importance is indicated by the degree to which parties view a relationship as critical to creating or sustaining their long-run competitive advantage. What is important to one partner in a relationship, however, may not be important to another. In characterizing the strategic importance of a relationship, it is necessary to reconcile and combine the different partners' perceptions or to create categories that allow for different assessments by each partner. In discussing hospital/physician relationships in this chapter, we generally adopt the hospital's perspective on the assessment of strategic purpose.

Our typology classifies relationships into four categories: firms (high strategic purpose, tight coupling), quasi firms (high strategic purpose, loose coupling), latent firms (low strategic purpose, tight coupling), and networks (low strategic purpose, loose coupling). At one extreme, then, are highly strategic, bureaucratic arrangements referred to as firms. At this extreme, interorganizational relationships become intraorganizational—the parts become a whole. At the other extreme are short-term, minor contractual links, with the lowest strategic purpose and least coupling, which are classified as network relationships. In between are quasi-firm and latent-firm arrangements.

Structural coupling between organizations and professionals, however, is not necessarily identical to the coupling that exists between organizations. Given the importance of autonomy in the definition of professionals as a category of worker, tight coupling per se may be difficult to achieve, at least functionally. Individual organizations can be assimilated within other organizations and thereby lose their identities. The same is not true for professionals. Although legal autonomy may be lost by professionals in employment relationships, functional autonomy usually is not, particularly for physicians. Tight coupling in organization/professional relationships, especially those involving physicians, may be a contradiction in terms. Scott recognized this contradiction (1982) in his conceptualization of hospital/physician structures. Although Scott identified heteronomous (hierarchical) structures, he recognized that these may not be easily maintained in professional organizations, given traditional requirements for professional autonomy. Relationships between organizations (rather than between organizations and professionals), however, do not face similar barriers of autonomy and thus can and do vary from the most tightly to the most loosely coupled forms.

In Figure 5.1, we convey this difference between organization/organization and organization/professional relationships by employing the term *conjoint firm* rather than *firm* to refer to the organization/professional relationship that is tightest in coupling and highest in strategic purpose. Although our usage does not correspond directly to Scott's (1982; 1987, p. 238) description of the "conjoint professional organization," we find the conjoint firm to be a useful summary label for organizational forms that attempt to incorporate formally autonomous professionals yet recognize their continued functional autonomy. Conceivably, Scott's (1982, 1987) notion of the heteronomous professional organization or Mintzberg's (1979, 1983) professional bureaucracy could be substituted in Figure 5.1 for the conjoint firm or could be added to the figure as representative of more tightly coupled organizational forms.

Some advantages of this typology are that it includes both structural and strategic dimensions of relationships; it can be used

**Figure 5.1. Characteristics and Form
of Organization/Professional Relationships.**

Tightness of Coupling

	High	Low
High	Conjoint firm	Quasi firm
Low	Latent conjoint firm	Network

Degree of Strategic Purpose (High / Low)

to characterize both intra- and interorganizational relationships; and it takes into account the role of the environment in shaping organization/professional relationships through the environment's impact on strategic interdependence. These advantages are illustrated next in a further application of the typology to current examples of hospital/physician relationships.

Patterns in Hospital/Physician Relationships

To describe hospital/physician relationships, a wide diversity must be encompassed. *Physician* may refer to an individual physician, a physician group, or the medical staff of a hospital as a whole. One physician may have multiple relationships with one hospital or multiple relationships with several hospitals. Some of these relationships may be intraorganizational, others interorganizational. Additionally, the medical staff of a hospital is not a homogeneous unit. Different types of nonphysicians are on many medical staffs (dentists, podiatrists, optometrists, psychologists, chiropractors, nurse practitioners), and different types of privileges are granted to each professional (probationary, active, consulting, courtesy). Medical staffs include a large number of providers, and some (for example, heavy admitters) are more strategically important to the hospital than others. We discuss medical staffs as singular entities for analytic purposes only.

In discussing hospital/medical-staff relationships later in the chapter, we generalize across several different types within the same hospital—for example, relationships involving clinical-quality management and those involving capital budgeting. In reality, different levels of strategic purpose and coupling may characterize different hospital/medical-staff relationships depending on the function of the relationship.

Another application issue, already noted, is reconciling different partners' perspectives on the degree of strategic purpose in a relationship. In this chapter, for simplification, we will consider hospital/physician relationships from the perspective of the hospital rather than the physician. The notion of a focal organization (in this case, the hospital) is common in the study of interorganizational relationships (Aldrich and Whetten, 1981; Morrissey, Hall, and Lindsey, 1982). Adopting the physician as the focal organization might result in alternative classifications of some relationships.

Classifications. We first use our typology to generalize about structure and strategy in relationships between hospitals and their medical staffs. Some hospital/medical-staff relationships are conjoint-firm relationships. An example is a staff-model health maintenance organization in a competitive environment, where virtually all the medical staff are salaried and medical-staff involvement is critical to the hospital's success. Another example might be teaching hospitals in competitive environments, where again the medical-staff members are full-time salaried, and physicians are a critical component of the hospital's strategic success. These types of hospital/physician relationships, while rare, come closest to the types of relationships found in other industries between organizations and professionals. For hospitals in this category, Mintzberg's (1979, 1983) professional-bureaucracy model, as well as the intraorganizational management-of-professionals literature cited previously, is likely to apply. However, the degree of strategic interdependence between organizations and professionals that distinguishes some professional bureaucracies from others is missing from Mintzberg's classification scheme.

Some hospital/medical-staff relationships may be characterized as tightly coupled but low on strategic purpose; these hospitals are latent conjoint firms. This classification would necessitate that the hospital consider its medical staff to be of low strategic importance, which in today's economic climate may be difficult. Perhaps coming closest to such a case are Veterans Administration hospitals and teaching hospitals that have captive patient bases and an abundant supply of physicians. Because physicians' work would not be critical in assuring the competitive advantage of these organizations, the degree of strategic purpose in the hospital/medical-staff relationship could be classified as low. However, the degree of shared strategic purpose could rise in time if competitive and financing pressures force these organizations to become strategically active. Such forms thus have a latent potential to emerge as actual conjoint firms.

The quasi-firm form includes hospitals whose relationships with their medical staff are strategically important, relatively permanent, and loosely coupled. This classification includes many community hospitals that operate in competitive settings but do not have tightly coupled relationships with their medical staffs. For such hospitals, the more competitive the market, the more likely that quasi-firm relationships exist. Those hospitals consider good hospital/physician relationships to be critical to their survival, but they deal with physicians (individually and collectively) as independent entities. Although relationships with physicians are perceived to be both permanent and important, physicians are not employees and have only a loosely coupled relationship with the hospitals in which they practice. In the most loosely coupled of the quasi-firm relationships, a separately incorporated medical staff is linked to the hospital only by a contractual agreement. While rare (McDermott, 1988), these arrangements conceptually are not very different from many existing arrangements (both are quasi-firm forms), and barriers to their implementation are largely legal and historical rather than conceptual.

Finally, some hospitals have a network relationship with their medical staffs. Our use of the term *network* here is different from its use in the health care literature to mean an aggregate of physicians under an organizational structure that maintains their functional autonomy and fee-for-service reimbursement, such as in an independent practice association (IPA) or preferred provider organization (PPO). We assign a general meaning to the term. In our typology, relationships between physicians and an IPA or PPO would be classified as either a network or a quasi firm depending on the strategic purpose of the arrangement. Although it is increasingly uncommon for a hospital to perceive its relationships with its medical staff to be low on strategic purpose, community hospitals that are sole providers in isolated market areas or that hold monopolistic positions in their major market areas may be better able to assign a low strategic priority to medical-staff relations than their counterparts in competitive environments. (This formulation would exclude hospitals that face a physician shortage and need to devote strategic attention to the recruitment and retention of physicians.) Creating competitive advantage through physician relationships is not as important a concern for such hospitals. Many may manage hospital/physician relationships as networks rather than as quasi firms. A hospital executive faced with managing a network rather than a quasi firm may give somewhat less attention, for example, to physician involvement in hospital strategic planning.

A wide range of relationships between hospitals and physicians exists in addition to medical-staff relationships. Joint ventures between hospitals and groups of physicians are common, with governance by contract or by joint organizations variously referred to as parallel organizations (Shortell, 1985), physician/hospital organizations (McManis, 1988), or medical-staff/hospital organizations (Anderson, 1985). These organizations typically create loosely coupled but formalized arrangements with varying levels of strategic purpose. Relationships that involve small-asset transactions for a specified outcome, typically investments by small groups of physicians, are likely to be lower in strategic purpose than large-asset transactions or transactions that involve significant commitments of physician time to pursue mutual goals. The less strategic activities are distinguished by some as microtransactions rather than macrotransactions ("Structuring Joint Hospital-Physician Ventures," 1988). Other examples of new forms of hospital/physician relationships are the sale of hospitals to physicians with a lease-back by the hospital (Uhlar, 1987) and hospital purchase of physician practices (Grayson, 1989), both events of high strategic importance. Of low strategic purpose are various types of new services provided by hospitals to physicians, such as new-practice setup, computerized physician links, and third-party claims processing (Belmont, 1988).

Trends. Some general patterns in the nature of hospital/physician relationships are evident. In the past, these relationships were generally of low strategic purpose (because developing competitive advantage through those relationships was not a major concern) and were loosely coupled; in other words, they were network relationships. Where physicians were employees of hospitals (and thus tightly coupled), relationships generally were still low in strategic purpose (latent conjoint firms).

Now and in the immediate future, hospital/physician relationships are and will be increasing in shared strategic purpose. A great deal of consensus exists that to create and sustain competitive advantage, permanent and strategically important relationships with physicians are a vital, if not the most vital, concern of hospital management (Berki, 1988; Bettner and Collins, 1987; Burns, 1986; Derzon, 1988; Goldsmith, 1989; McDermott, 1988; McManis, 1988; Shortell, Morrison, Friedman, and associates, 1989). For example, joint ventures between hospitals and physicians are described in the following terms by one leading health care executive in the preface to a book on that topic: "Even though viewed by some as only a stage in [the] development of an integrated health system, joint ventures must be viewed as long-term relationships that, if successful, will build a base of confidence, working relationship, professional incentive, and financial interdependence which will serve as a positive base for future developments. . . . This book speaks clearly about the need for a long-term view and structure for hospital-physician joint ventures." (D.C. Wegmiller, in Burns and Mancino, 1987, pp. vii–viii). Joint ventures are viewed in this passage as both relatively permanent and high in strategic importance. Even a hospital-sponsored physician computer network is touted as a key strategy for hospital survival (Tiedemann, 1987).

Although increasing in strategic purpose, hospital/physi-

cian relationships still often remain loosely coupled. Hospital tactics such as joint ventures, adding physician liaison staff or physician board members, and developing physician bonding programs
speak more to the increasing strategic importance of the hospital/
physician relationship than they do to modifying the tightness of
the coupling between the two. Although hospitals may appear, in
some cases, to be increasing the tightness of coupling with physicians, the need to preserve traditional professional autonomy may
channel such tightening through the strategic rather than the structural dimension.

The deprofessionalization and proletarianization literature
(for example, McKinlay and Arches, 1985) argues that all hospital/
physician relationships are moving in the direction of tighter coupling and governance by heteronomous or conjoint firms, as physicians begin to be treated like other employees, but there is a
substantial body of contrary opinion (for example, Freidson, 1985;
Hafferty, 1988). Experimentation with managed health care systems
suggests a willingness to try bureaucratic mechanisms to increase
the level of control over physical practice. However, bureaucratic
controls can be expected to be resisted by physicians, leaving the
market-modified version of the conjoint model as a likely alternative. Although physicians clearly are sacrificing some degree of autonomy in nontechnical zones, their control of the technical zone
(Freidson, 1970, p. 45) has not been significantly altered. As a result,
it is likely that even as hospital/physician relationships become
increasingly tight and strategically important, the form of that relationship at its extreme will resemble a conjoint firm rather than
a traditional business firm.

A diversity of strategically important organizational forms is
thus emerging in the health care sector. Many hospital efforts to
collaborate with physicians for competitive advantage fall into the
quasi-firm category. Because of the recent emergence (or recognition) of quasi-firm arrangements in the health care marketplace and
the fact that management issues in the quasi firm are unexplored
(especially relative to conjoint firms or professional bureaucracies),
in the remainder of the chapter we focus on the distinctive management issues that arise in such arrangements.

Managing Quasi-Firm Relationships
Between Hospitals and Physicians

Quasi-firm relationships are probably the most difficult types of relationships to manage because the stakes are high (strategic purpose is high) and because loose coupling requires more subtle management skills and fewer direct controls than tight coupling. Quasi-firm relationships between hospitals and physicians often are replete with paradoxes for hospital managers—for example, how does the hospital collaborate with physicians in the quasi-firm relationship yet simultaneously compete with the same physicians in other relationships? Elsewhere, we have argued that four managerial tasks are particularly prominent and problematical in the quasi firm: balancing flexibility and stability, making strategic decisions, ensuring a unified effort by members, and determining and modifying the boundaries of the quasi firm (Luke, Begun, and Pointer, 1989). These tasks resemble the four key issues identified by Borys and Jemison (1989) in their discussion of new organizational combinations: breadth of purpose, boundary determination, (joint) value creation, and stability.

These issues as they typically arise in hospital/physician arrangements are briefly examined next. All are based on the fact that each member of a loosely coupled arrangement is likely to be responsive to some unique forces not affecting other quasi-firm members. Although loose coupling promotes the formation of the quasi firm in the first place and hopefully abets its permanence, it is also a built-in source of goal incompatibility and potential conflict among the partners. Given the strategic nature of the quasi firm, efforts to overcome these disadvantages become critical to competitive success. Hospital executives accustomed to managing network relationships in the past may find it necessary to devote time and resources to focusing on the distinctive management issues of the quasi-firm relationship. Successful quasi-firm management is likely to require difficult and carefully weighed decisions by hospital executives—for example, about which physicians to invest in, how to sanction low performers, and how much hospital autonomy to sacrifice, all issues that were much simpler or nonexistent in the not-so-distant past.

Balancing Flexibility and Stability. Flexibility is a major advantage of the quasi firm. Members are able to pursue diverse goals, some of which may be incompatible with those of other quasi-firm members. Like firms, however, quasi firms can be expected to attempt to reduce uncertainty and create stability through tighter coupling. Pressures to tighten coupling in the quasi firm are likely to be higher in environments that are relatively uncertain than in those that are not because loose coupling may provide insufficient cohesiveness for collectives to be able to respond quickly to environmental shifts (Bresser and Harl, 1986). Stability can be created in the quasi firm through the use of long-term contracts, the development of trust, or reliance on shared industry norms (Borys and Jemison, 1989).

The building of trust between hospitals and physicians in today's health care market may be unlikely, as physicians and hospitals do not share a common set of norms about business practices. Thus, a reservoir of trust that has already been developed, based on years of experience, is a distinct advantage to the hospital/physician quasi firm. Empirically, we would expect hospital/physician organizations that are built on a significant foundation of trust to outperform others.

Pressures to stabilize may be counterproductive if they lead to abandonment of the quasi-firm form. For instance, success in important collaborative efforts might cause quasi-firm members to merge formally, thus jeopardizing important assets of the quasi-firm relationship. Merged partners may find themselves in a permanent relationship they may come to regret. The problems encountered when hospitals purchase physician group practices may be an example of this issue.

At the same time, the different goals of the partners in a quasi firm often result in pressures to loosen coupling, even to the point of destroying the quasi firm. For example, hospital managers may lose interest in a successful joint venture with one physician group if a different joint venture promises even better results for the hospital. At the least, such developments reduce both trust and the commitment of a partner to the arrangement.

Making Strategic Decisions. Quasi firms are faced with the need to make new strategic decisions as circumstances change, particularly in volatile environments, and therefore a strategic decision-making and implementation apparatus must exist. Certain members of the quasi firm must have more decision-making power than others, particularly when quick decisions are needed. In hospital/physician relationships, hospitals can often claim greater prior experience with and existing administrative support for strategic decision making than physicians, arguing for greater hospital control of the process. In fact, many activities labeled as hospital/physician joint ventures may be more properly labeled as internal joint ventures by hospitals, with equity participation by hospitals and physicians but staffing provided by a unit linked closely to the hospital (Shortell and Zajac, 1988). However, such hospital control may endanger the commitment of physicians to the quasi firm unless countered by time-consuming communication and consensus building. A major alternative, equal representation in strategic decision making, may lead to stalemates. Inviting third parties into the quasi firm is a potential solution (McDermott, 1988).

Ensuring Unified Effort. Building unity of effort in the quasi firm requires time and attention, although comprehensive information systems and exchange of information can substitute for lengthy trust-building processes (Miles and Snow, 1986). Developing internal cohesion and trust is more critical in the quasi firm than the firm because of the relative inability to sanction and control members. In hospital/physician organizations, physicians frequently are skeptical of the motives of hospital management. And because most hospital/physician quasi firms are relatively new, the reluctance of physicians and hospitals to trust each other is strong. In addition, hospital personnel often have no experience with physician relationships or are perceived as biased, necessitating that independent staff be hired. Consistency across type of relationship and consistency over time would contribute to the development of trust and cohesion on both sides of the hospital/physician relationship.

Determining and Modifying Boundaries. Admission requirements for existing and ongoing quasi firms, and methods for the expulsion or sanctioning of members, are the final dimensions of organization that require special attention in the quasi firm. Because the choice of "right" partners is important in developing trust (Jarillo, 1988), creating and modifying boundaries are particularly critical issues. Many quasi firms, hoping to avoid the issue, probably do not have well-specified procedures for sanctioning members. Legal and ethical constraints on joint activities by hospitals and physicians, however, affect the resolution of this question by discouraging physicians from referring patients to facilities in which they have a financial stake (American Medical Association, 1986).

All these issues, while facing managers of firms as well as quasi firms, are particularly problematic in quasi-firm management. They pose new dilemmas for health care executives and require new interorganizational management skills. The empirical experience of new hospital/physician organizations in resolving these issues will be a source of new insights into the management of organization/professional relationships.

Implications for Other Industries and for Research

We have argued that one important reality of organizational forms is that their structure and strategy are separately important and that classification of these forms should be based jointly on structure and strategy. We have found it useful to treat the physician as an organization and to classify hospital/physician relationships as conjoint firms, latent conjoint firms, quasi firms, and networks.

Classification of a relationship as a quasi firm leads one to focus on certain managerial issues: creating stability without destroying flexibility, designing strategic decision processes, unifying efforts, and determining boundaries. We have suggested that hospital managers devote increased attention to these issues as they develop the multitude of hospital/physician arrangements emerging in the health care market today.

Generalizing to Other Industries. Designing and managing relationships with professionals have been viewed as intraorganizational tasks in most industries. Most organization/professional relationships have been (implicitly) perceived as either conjoint firms or latent conjoint firms. Coupling is tighter, and relationships less strategically important, than is true for most hospital/physician relationships. The literature on professionals in bureaucracies, referred to previously, is relevant to understanding and managing these relationships. These relationships include professors in universities, engineers in construction firms, research and development personnel in manufacturing firms, and lawyers in legal firms. Our specific discussion of quasi-firm management, then, may have limited utility for organization/professional relationships in other industries.

However, the quasi-firm image may be useful to organizations interested in reaping the benefits of increased autonomy for professional workers. Where innovation is strategically important, for instance, quasi-firm relationships can provide important incentives to professionals who historically have been managed through firm or conjoint-firm configurations. Joint ventures between universities and groups of faculty members to develop biogenetic agents and computer hardware and software are an example, as are some relationships between private research-and-development organizations and research scientists. The equivalent of hospital/physician organizations could be created in other industries in order to stimulate innovation by professionals.

For example, a strong case could be made that the relationship between universities and their faculty members is becoming increasingly like the relationship between hospitals and physicians. Universities, like hospitals, are facing increasing pressures to economize internally, to compete for inputs (students), and to be innovative in order to generate new resources. In addition, they traditionally have maintained a dual line of authority, with professors having a high degree of (at least functional) autonomy. We might characterize the university as moving from being a latent conjoint firm to being a conjoint firm, with relationships between universities and their faculties (relatively) tightly coupled and important for competitive success. As joint strategic purpose increases, we can expect universities to apply approaches suited to managing conjoint firms, such as team building, conflict resolution, and joint decision making.

Consider, however, an alternative: that universities develop quasi firms, with far looser coupling between professors and administrators, at least for purposes of developing innovative teaching and research programs. University-faculty organizations governed jointly by the university and teaching or research professionals, could undertake speculative applied-research programs or market new teaching programs—for example, electronic network classes for full-time workers or teleconferences. Centralized services, such as those of the university library, could be purchased by the quasi firm. The quasi-firm organizations could compete with traditional conjoint-firm arrangements in the same way that varying forms of hospital/physician organizations do in the health care sector.

Research Issues. The emergence of interorganizational forms other than fully integrated firms to govern organization/professional relationships raises new research issues. Although several conceptual issues have been broached, virtually no empirical research is available, and thus a broad range of opportunities exists.

A first requirement is that the identification and classification of organization/professional relationships be further addressed. Classification dimensions other than degree of coupling and strategic purpose may be important. For instance, the directionality of relationships, which can be vertical, horizontal, or symbiotic, may influence the choice of governing form. Borys and Jemison (1989) make a strong case for the importance of the type of interdependence (pooled, sequential, or reciprocal) among members of a hybrid arrangement. Quasi-firm control in the most complex form of interdependence, reciprocal, no doubt takes longer to evolve and requires greater flexibility in initial arrangements than control in the other two forms. Beyond the conceptual issues, how are differences in strategic purpose and coupling best measured? What is the distribution of values on these variables across populations of hospital/physician relationships? How common is the quasi firm compared with the conjoint firm?

A second area for research is the empirical study of management issues that arise in quasi-firm and conjoint-firm relationships. What governance, decision-making, and reward structures characterize existing relationships between hospitals and physicians? How are nonperformers sanctioned? How is performance monitored? How stable is membership over time? Answers to such questions would lead to improved operational understanding of conjoint firms and quasi firms and improved counsel for managers working with such firms.

An issue related to these management questions is that in a volatile environment we anticipate a high degree of movement between the different organizational forms. We have argued that as environments become more uncertain, organizations may use either market (quasi-firm) or bureaucratic (conjoint-firm) mechanisms to resolve increased pressures to achieve control over the work of professionals. Patterns in the transition of forms no doubt exist, and the impact of environmental characteristics on the choice and transition of forms may be especially interesting.

Finally, one could explore differences in organization/professional relationships across professions and across organizational types. For example, what differences exist between specialty hospitals and general hospitals in the degree of strategic purpose and coupling in their relationships with physicians? Between hospital/physician relationships and hospital/nurse and other clinical-provider relationships? Between hospital/physician and legal-firm/lawyer relationships? Such questions might redirect studies of professionals to include the strategic dimension of relationships with organizations. Relationships characterized by high shared strategic purpose, we have argued, will be quite different from those with low strategic purpose.

In this chapter we have modified a typology previously developed for interorganizational relationships and applied it to hospital/physician relationships. The reality of health care delivery is such that it is fruitful for hospitals to treat physicians as strategically interdependent business firms, either incorporating them into conjoint-firm arrangements or dealing with them in quasi-firm relationships. The diverse, new organizational landscape in the health care industry no doubt will continue to reflect the growing strategic interdependence between hospitals and physicians.

References

Aldrich, H., and Whetten, D. A. "Organization-Sets, Action-Sets, and Networks: Making the Most of Simplicity." In P. C. Nystrom and W. H. Starbuck (eds.), *Handbook of Organizational Design.* Vol. 1. New York: Oxford University Press, 1981.

Alexander, J. A., Morrisey, M. A., and Shortell, S. M. "Effects of Competition, Regulation, and Corporatization on Hospital-Physician Relationships." *Journal of Health and Social Behavior,* 1986, *27,* 220–235.

American Medical Association. *Physician-Hospital Joint Ventures: A Resource Manual for Physicians and Physician Advisers.* Chicago: American Medical Association, 1986.

Anderson, J. G. "The MeSH Model for Hospital-Physician Joint Ventures." *Health Matrix,* 1985, *3* (1), 32–37.

Astley, W. G. "Toward an Appreciation of Collective Strategy." *Academy of Management Review,* 1984, *9,* 526–535.

Astley, W. G., and Fombrun, C. J. "Collective Strategy: Social Ecology of Organizational Environments." *Academy of Management Review,* 1983, *8,* 576–587.

Belmont, T. A. "Use Joint Ventures to Strengthen Hospital/MD Relationships." *Trustee,* 1988, *41* (1), 17, 19.

Benveniste, G. *Professionalizing the Organization.* San Francisco: Jossey-Bass, 1987.

Berki, S. E. "Changes in Hospital-Doctor Relations." *Consultant,* 1988, *28* (2), 114–116, 119.

Bettner, M., and Collins, F. "Physicians and Administrators: Inducing Collaboration." *Hospital and Health Services Administration,* 1987, *32* (2), 151–160.

Borys, B., and Jemison, D. B. "Hybrid Arrangements as Strategic Alliances: Theoretical Issues in Organizational Combinations." *Academy of Management Review,* 1989, *14* (2), 234–249.

Bresser, R., and Harl, J. "Collective Strategy: Vice or Virtue?" *Academy of Management Review,* 1986, *11,* 408–427.

Burchell, R. C., White, R. E., Smith, H. L., and Piland, N. F. "Physicians and the Organizational Evolution of Medicine." *Journal of the American Medical Association,* 1988, *260* (6), 826–831.

Burns, L. A., and Mancino, D. M. *Joint Ventures Between Hospitals and Physicians: A Competitive Strategy for the Healthcare Marketplace.* Homewood, Ill.: Dow Jones-Irwin, 1987.

Burns, L. R. "Hospital-Medical Staff Tensions: An Historical Overview and Analysis." *Journal of Medical Practice Management,* 1986, *1* (3), 191-198.

Derzon, R. A. "The Odd Couple in Distress: Hospitals and Physicians Face the 1990s." *Frontiers of Health Services Management,* 1988, *4* (3), 4-19.

Freidson, E. *Profession of Medicine: A Study of the Sociology of Applied Knowledge.* New York: Dodd, Mead, 1970.

Freidson, E. "The Reorganization of the Medical Profession." *Medical Care Review,* 1985, *42* (1), 11-35.

Freidson, E. *Professional Powers: A Study of the Institutionalization of Formal Knowledge.* Chicago: University of Chicago Press, 1986.

Glandon, G. L., and Morrisey, M. A. "Redefining the Hospital-Physician Relationship Under Prospective Payment." *Inquiry,* 1986, *23,* 166-175.

Glassman, R. B. "Persistence and Loose Coupling in Living Systems." *Behavioral Science,* 1973, *18,* 83-98.

Goldsmith, J. "A Radical Prescription for Hospitals." *Harvard Business Review,* 1989, *89* (3), 104-111.

Grayson, M. A. "Breaking the Medical Gridlock." *Hospitals,* 1989, *63* (4), 32-37.

Griffith, J. R. *The Well-Managed Community Hospital.* Ann Arbor, Mich.: Health Administration Press, 1987.

Hafferty, F. W. "Theories at the Crossroads: A Discussion of Evolving Views on Medicine as a Profession." *The Milbank Quarterly,* 1988, *66* (supp. 2), 202-225.

Harris, J. E. "The Internal Organization of Hospitals: Some Economic Implications." *Bell Journal of Economics,* 1977, *8,* 467-482.

Herbert-Carter, J. "Cooperative Coordination: A New Style of Health Care Administration." *Health Matrix,* 1988, *6* (2), 56-65.

Jarillo, J. C. "On Strategic Networks." *Strategic Management Journal,* 1988, *9,* 31-41.

Kanter, R. M. *When Giants Learn to Dance: Mastering the Chal-*

lenges of Strategy, Management, and Careers in the 1990s. New York: Simon & Schuster, 1989.

Katz, R. (ed.). *Managing Professionals in Innovative Organizations.* Cambridge, Mass.: Ballinger, 1988.

Luke, R. D., Begun, J. W., and Pointer, D. D. "Quasi Firms: Strategic Interorganizational Forms in the Health Care Industry." *Academy of Management Review,* 1989, *14* (1), 9–19.

McDermott, S. "The New Hospital Challenge: Organizing and Managing Physician Organizations." *Health Care Management Review,* 1988, *13* (1), 57–61.

McKinlay, J. B., and Arches, J. "Towards the Proletarianization of Physicians." *International Journal of Health Services,* 1985, *15* (2), 161–195.

McManis, G. L. "If You Can't Beat 'Em, Join 'Em? The New Generation of PHOs." *Healthcare Executive,* 1988, *3* (5), 42.

Miles, R. E., and Snow, C. C. "Organizations: New Concepts for New Forms." *California Management Review,* 1986, *28* (3), 62–73.

Miller, J. G. *Living Systems.* New York: McGraw-Hill, 1978.

Mills, P. K., Hall, J. L., Leidecker, J. K., and Margulies, N. "Flexiform: A Model for Professional Service Organizations." *Academy of Management Review,* 1983, *8* (1), 118–131.

Mintzberg, H. *The Structuring of Organizations.* Englewood Cliffs, N.J.: Prentice-Hall, 1979.

Mintzberg, H. *Structure in Fives: Designing Effective Organizations.* Englewood Cliffs, N.J.: Prentice-Hall, 1983.

Mintzberg, H. "The Strategy Concept I: Five Ps for Strategy." In G. R. Carroll and D. Vogel (eds.), *Organizational Approaches to Strategy.* Cambridge, Mass.: Ballinger, 1987.

Morgan, G. *Images of Organization.* Beverly Hills, Calif.: Sage, 1986.

Morrissey, J. P., Hall, R. H., and Lindsey, M. L. *Interorganizational Relations: A Sourcebook of Measures for Mental Health Programs.* Department of Health and Human Services Publication (ADM) 82-1187. Washington, D.C.: U.S. Government Printing Office, 1982.

Pauly, M., and Redisch, M. "The Not-for-Profit Hospital as a Physicians' Cooperative." *American Economic Review*, 1973, *63* (1), 87–99.

Pointer, D. D., Begun, J. W., and Luke, R. D. "Managing Interorganizational Dependencies in the New Health Care Marketplace." *Hospital and Health Services Administration*, 1988, *33* (2), 167–177.

Powell, W. W. "Hybrid Organizational Arrangements: New Form or Transitional Development?" In G. R. Carroll and D. Vogel (eds.), *Organizational Approaches to Strategy*. Cambridge, Mass.: Ballinger, 1987.

Raelin, J. *The Clash of Cultures: Managers and Professionals*. Boston: Harvard Business School Press, 1986.

Rakich, J. S., Longest, B. B., and Darr, K. *Managing Health Services Organizations*. (2nd ed.) Philadephia: Saunders, 1985.

Scott, W. R. "Managing Professional Work: Three Models of Control for Health Organizations." *Health Services Research*, 1982, *17*, 213–240.

Scott, W. R. *Organizations: Rational, Natural, and Open Systems*. (2nd ed.) Englewood Cliffs, N.J.: Prentice-Hall, 1987.

Sheldon, A. *Managing Doctors*. Homewood, Ill.: Dow Jones-Irwin, 1986.

Shortell, S. M. "The Medical Staff of the Future." *Frontiers of Health Services Management*, 1985, *1* (3), 3–48.

Shortell, S. M., Morrison, E. M., Friedman, B., and associates. *America's Hospital Systems: Lessons in Managing Strategic Adaptation*. San Francisco: Jossey-Bass, 1989.

Shortell, S. M., and Zajac, E. J. "Internal Corporate Joint Ventures: Development Processes and Performance Outcomes." *Strategic Management Journal*, 1988, *9*, 527–542.

Smith, H. L. "Two Lines of Authority Are One Too Many." *Modern Hospital*, 1955, *84* (3), 59–64.

"Structuring Joint Hospital-Physician Ventures." *Hospital Entrepreneurs Newsletter*, 1988, *3* (8), 5–7.

Thorelli, H. B. "Networks: Between Markets and Hierarchies." *Strategic Management Journal*, 1986, *7*, 37–51.

Tiedemann, F. "Managing the Hospital/Physician Relationship: The Network as a Strategy for Survival." *Journal of Health Care Marketing*, 1987, *7* (3), 73–77.

Uhlar, B. "Sale/Lease-Back with Doctors Being Explored by Hospitals." *Hospitals,* 1987, *61* (4), 44.

Weick, K. E. "Educational Organizations as Loosely Coupled Systems." *Administrative Science Quarterly,* 1976, *21,* 1–19.

Williamson, O. E. *Markets and Hierarchies: Analysis and Antitrust Implications.* New York: Free Press, 1975.

6

Health Care Organizations and the Development of the Strategic-Management Perspective

Stephen M. Shortell
Edward J. Zajac

The rapidity and pervasiveness of changes occurring within the American health care system are widely acknowledged. For students of organizations, these changes have four important implications. The first is the need to examine the process by which organizations within an industry transform themselves to meet the demands of a radically new environment. The second is the need to expand concepts of organizational effectiveness based on a few stakeholders (for example, physicians and patients) to include a broad array of diverse stakeholders (for example, third-party payers, large employers, regulatory bodies, and legal and licensing agencies). The third is the need to change the primary focus of analysis from internal operations and performance to the organization's relationships to external stakeholders and its environment. The fourth implication is the need to move beyond the study of individual health care organizations to the study of strategic alliances involving systems or networks of health care organizations. In addressing these issues, research on health care organizations has generally kept pace with parallel developments in the organizational sciences at large and, in a few cases, may even be at the cutting edge.

In this chapter we provide a brief overview of strategic-management theory and the contributions of health care organizational research to that theory. The main focus, however, is on two subareas of investigation: strategic change and adaptation, and the development of strategic alliances. These areas are selected because of their importance both to the health care sector and to the study of strategy in general. In each area we draw on recent research to illustrate its potential contributions for further theory development.

The State of Strategic-Management Theory

Strategic-management theory has its origin in Chandler's (1962) seminal work on strategy and structure. This work is reinforced by the conceptual work of Ansoff (1965), Andrews (1971), and Schendel and Hofer (1979), and more recently by Porter's insights into competitive strategy (1980, 1985). Although disagreements exist in the literature about what should be included in the defintion of strategy—some favoring a broad definition that includes the goals and objectives of the firm (Chandler, 1962; Andrews, 1971) and others favoring a narrow definition limited to the plans and activities of the organization (Ansoff, 1965; Schendel and Hofer, 1979)—all agree that strategy involves positioning the organization relative to its environment and competitors in order to achieve its goals and assure its survival. This formulation of strategy has led to two main streams of investigation: issues and questions of strategic content, and issues and questions of strategic process. The content research has focused primarily on the relationship among the firm's strategies, its environment, and its performance. It has addressed issues of diversification, generic-strategy taxonomies, strategic groups, and the evolution of markets, among other topics (Fahey and Christensen, 1986). The process-oriented research has focused on issues of strategy formulation and implementation. Attention has been paid to planning methods, decision-making processes, the alignment of strategy and structure, and their effects on performance (Huff and Reger, 1987).

Ansoff (1987) has suggested the emergence of a paradigm centered around the idea that the strategic behavior of an organization should be examined as a function of the interplay among environmental forces, internal organizational configurations and processes, and strategic content. Along similar lines, Kimberly and Zajac (1985) call for an examination of the connections among environment/strategy, strategy/structure, and structure/behavior. These approaches attempt to integrate strategic-content and strategic-process research while taking into account the nature of the organization's relationship to its environment.

For further progress to be made, however, it is necessary to address several issues and questions that have received relatively little attention in either the content or process literature to date. Among these are:

- The role strategy plays in achieving the nonfinancial goals of the organization, particularly in regard to diverse stakeholder groups. Almost without exception, the current literature is focused on accounting and financial indicators as measures of the success of a firm's strategy.
- Examination of the conditions under which some firms are likely to change their strategy and which types of strategic change are more likely than others to be effective.
- Emerging cooperative strategies and strategic alliances that go beyond the current preoccupation with a single firm's competitive strategies.
- Studies that explore in depth the relationship between the corporate office and the division in the strategy-making process of multidivisional organizations.
- What happens in the strategy formulation and implementation process when power bases are diffuse and when key leaders lack formal position, power, or authority.
- Examination of the extent to which strategy formulation and implementation are intertwined processes and the conditions under which strategies are likely to be generated out of the implementation process rather than formulated in advance.
- Further investigation of the role of internal transaction costs and benefits in strategy implementation and performance.

Health care is a particularly attractive area for addressing these issues. Because of the broad mission of most health care organizations and the fact that the industry is composed of both for-profit and not-for-profit firms, a wide range of performance issues (both financial and nonfinancial) can be addressed. In addition, one can examine the extent to which the objectives of a diverse array of stakeholders are met. Given the significant changes occurring within the industry, it also serves as a fertile ground for examining the extent to which organizations change their strategies, the conditions under which certain strategies are more effective than others, and the process by which new strategies are successfully implemented. It also provides an opportunity for observing the implementation of cooperative strategies (for example, strategic alliances and networks) and of acquisition and divestment strategies (for example, hospital and clinical as well as support service consolidations and closings). The growth of hospital systems affords excellent opportunities for studying various aspects of the corporate office/division relationship, ranging from strategic-planning processes to the centralization versus decentralization of decision making to transaction-cost economics.

In addition to these content issues, the health care sector also serves as a laboratory for examining process-oriented issues. For example, the prominent role played by diverse groups of health care professionals opens up new opportunities for studying the nature of strategic planning and implementation. How are these processes conducted when power among key actors is dispersed and when members of one of the key groups (physicians) are usually not even employees of the organization? Health care organizations also can provide rich insights into the growing normative assertion that strategy formulation and implementation are highly interrelated processes because a health care organization's ability to implement many of its strategies depends on early and significant involvement of physicians and other key professional groups. The diffuse power base along with the rapidity of change also provide opportunities for studying the relationship between formal and informal planning and between induced and autonomous planning (Burgelman, 1987).

Current Research

The push for an economical and cost-effective health care system means that organizations must consider health care as both an economic and a social good. To learn how these different ideologies are balanced requires an explicit examination of the strategies pursued by health care organizations and the processes by which they are formulated, implemented, and evaluated (Kimberly and Zajac, 1985; Shortell, Morrison, and Robbins, 1985).

A small but growing literature has emerged that addresses the strategic behavior of health care organizations and provides some insights into the development of strategic-management theory at large. A sample of relevant conceptual and empirical work from the 1980s is highlighted in Figure 6.1. Works are classified according to the content categories suggested by Kimberly and Zajac (1985). Although there is reasonable coverage of each category, empirical examination of the connections among the three categories has only begun.

Longest's (1981) resource-dependence perspective on the strategy-making process gives a prominent role to the organization's leaders as the "key strategists." They are charged with the responsibility for perceiving the environment and aligning the organization's distinctive competence with the demands of the environment. The important role played by the top-management team in the strategy-making process is only beginning to appear in the strategic-management literature (Hambrick and Finkelstein, 1987). Further research on health care organizational leadership can make an important contribution to understanding the top-management team's role in the overall strategy-making process.

Longest also emphasizes that implementation is influenced by a complex interplay of strategies, tasks, structures, technologies, and people; relatively little is known about this process. A major question that emerges is the extent to which implementation can be or should be structured through the formal strategic-planning process or left fluid. Burgelman (1987) takes up this issue by contrasting the role played by induced (structured) versus autonomous (fluid) approaches in the process of strategic adaptation.

The work of Peters and Tseng (1983) and Shortell, Morrison, and Friedman (1990) highlights some of the behavioral dynamics associated with strategic adaptation. They emphasize the importance of five factors: the role of precipitators of change—events or circumstances that make the status quo uncomfortable; the need to articulate desired alternative states; the importance of the organiza-

**Figure 6.1. Classification of Selected Health Care
Organizational-Research Contributions to Strategic-Management Theory**

Environment/Strategy	*Strategy/Structure*	*Structure/Behavior*
(C) Longest (1981) ──────────────────────────────────▶		
	(E) Peters and Tseng (1983) ─────────────▶	
	(E) Shortell, Wickizer, and Wheeler (1984) ──────▶	
(C) Kimberly and Zajac (1985) ─────────────────────────▶		
(C) Shortell, Morrison, and Robbins (1985) ────────────▶		
	(E) Clement (1987)	
	(E) Alexander, Morlock, and Gifford (1988)	
(E) Keats, Conant, and Mokwa (1988)		
	(E) Luke and Begun (1988)	
	(C) Mick and Conrad (1988) ──────────▶	
(E) Shortell and Zajac (1988) ─────────────────────────▶		
(E) Zajac and Shortell (1989)		
(E) Ginn (1990)		
(E) Zajac, Golden, and Shortell (1990) ────────────────▶		
(E) Shortell, Morrison, and Friedman (1990) ───────────▶		

Note: C = conceptual, E = empirical.

tion's culture and value system in successfully initiating such change; the need to take risks; and the need to manage the timing and pace of change. In studying the problems associated with the implementation of one strategy—hospital/physician joint ventures involving primary-care group practices—Shortell, Wickizer, and Wheeler (1984) and Shortell and Zajac (1988) highlight the importance of balancing autonomy needs and integration needs in structuring relationships between the parent organization and new units. Zajac, Golden, and Shortell (1990) also discuss the role of such relationships in enhancing innovation. These findings have added to a growing literature on new venture developments and organizational spinoffs.

The conceptual pieces of Kimberly and Zajac (1985) and Shortell, Morrison, and Robbins (1985) lay out a number of issues, questions, and hypotheses requiring attention. Subsequent work has addressed some of these areas. The most productive stream of research (Ginn, 1990) has been that examining the changes in the health care environment and strategic content, particularly in reference to Miles and Snow's (1978) typology of prospectors (consistently innovative), analyzers (market niche oriented), defenders (protective of current domains), and reactors (lacking a consistent strategy) (Keats, Conant, and Mokwa, 1988; Luke and Begun, 1988; Zajac and Shortell, 1989; Shortell, Morrison, and Friedman, 1990). Most of these studies (Luke and Begun did not examine performance) have found generally consistent findings pertaining to the degree of strategic change initiated by health care organizations— approximately 38 to 50 percent in various samples; the direction of change—from a defender orientation to an analyzer and prospector orientation; the importance of prior strategy in initiating strategic change; and the general superior performance of organizations adopting an analyzer or prospector strategy versus those adopting a defender or reactor strategy. Shortell, Morrison, and Friedman (1990) examine some of the underlying factors that account for these findings, including the requirements for managing the different strategic orientations. This stream of health care organzational research has made important contributions to the strategic-management literature at large by suggesting that in turbulent environments a proactive analyzer or prospector strategy appears to be preferable to a defender or reactor strategy and is associated with superior performance. The health care organizational literature also provides some empirical data relevant to the frequency with which firms change strategies and the direction in which those changes occur.

Other work noted in Table 6.1 has examined the effects of

specific strategies or structural elements. For example, Clement's (1987) data indicate that diversification has not paid off for most hospitals, although more recent research suggests some of the factors that may distinguish the more successful diversifiers from the less successful (Shortell, Morrison, and Hughes, 1989). Alexander, Morlock, and Gifford (1988) document how hospital restructuring has resulted in corporation-like hospital boards rather than philanthropic boards and a consequent increase in the strategic orientation of such boards. Mick and Conrad (1988) provide useful guidelines for considering vertical-integration strategies based on Williamson's (1975) transaction-cost perspective. Of particular note is the emphasis they give to internal behavioral impediments such as goal displacement, poor communication, and poor conflict resolution, which can increase "internal" transaction costs.

Strategic Adaptation

In a world in which change is common and continuity uncommon, the study of strategic adaptation is of particular importance. It also provides a lens for studying many organizational phenomena because it is under conditions of change that new issues and processes arise, underlying assumptions are exposed, and new insights are uncovered. Among the more important and interesting aspects of strategic change are the prevalence, direction, magnitude, pace, duration, and effects of the process. In particular we are interested in the circumstances (external and internal to the organization) surrounding the process. For example, under what circumstances and conditions do organizations change or not change their strategies? Two studies of strategic change in health care organizations specifically address some of these issues. They provide a departure point for developing an integrative framework to guide future theory development and testing.

Prevalence of Change. Using different samples of hospitals, both Ginn (1990) and Zajac and Shortell (1989) observed strategic changes (as measured by the Miles and Snow typology of prospectors, analyzers, defenders, and reactors) to occur with some frequency—in 38 percent of the 77 Texas hospitals studied by Ginn from 1976 to 1980 and from 1981 to 1985, and in 54 percent of 510 hospitals belonging to eight hospital systems nationwide studied by Zajac and Shortell from 1983 to 1985. Subsequent work indicates that 50 percent of system hospitals changed their strategic orientations between 1985 and 1987 (Shortell, Morrison and Friedman, 1990). Both Ginn and Zajac and Shortell found that prior strategy (specifically, being a defender) was the strongest predictor of the probability of a change in strategic orientation. These findings suggest that, at least in industries or sectors undergoing significant environmental turmoil, organizations are more likely to change their strategies than is suggested by some of the literature (for example, Hannan and Freeman, 1984). The failure to observe a greater prevalence or frequency of strategic change in the past may be due to the selection of industries that were relatively stable.

Direction of Change. Ginn (1990), Zajac and Shortell (1989), and Shortell, Morrison, and Friedman (1990) all find a consistent shift in strategy from the more passive defender category to the more active analyzer and prospector categories. It appears that not all strategies are equally preferred for given environmental states. In the face of significant environmental change, active market-oriented responses involving the analyzer and prospector approaches are favored. This response appears to be due to the belief that the organization needs to develop new products or services (needs to diversify) to compete in new markets; in the case of health care, these new services and products include outpatient diagnostic centers, home health care, and sports medicine. In this way, a hospital can both protect the acute-care business and develop new revenue sources.

Magnitude of Change. If one accepts the Miles and Snow (1978) continuum of the defender strategy as the least change-oriented and the prospector strategy as the most change-oriented, then the magnitude of switching from a defender to a prospector strategy would be greater than that of switching from a defender to an analyzer or an analyzer to a prospector. In Ginn's (1990) work, of the seventeen defenders who switched their strategies, five became reactors, eight became analyzers, while only four became prospectors. Of the four analyzers who switched strategies, two became prospectors and two reactors; none became a defender. All four of the prospectors who switched strategies became analyzers. These results suggest that hospitals seldom move more than one category away from their base orientation on the Miles and Snow strategic continuum.

These results are confirmed by national studies finding that 65 percent of all strategic changes were made within adjacent categories (Shortell, Morrison, and Friedman, 1990). The authors suggest that this observation might be explained by the notion of a strategic comfort zone within which organizations wish to operate even when recognizing the need for a significant degree of strategic reorientation. The idea of the strategic comfort zone involves the extent to which the new strategy requires a significant departure from the organization's current culture, values, behavioral norms, practices, policies, and mix of abilities and skills. In brief, to what extent does the organization feel comfortable about the new strategy and capable of implementing it? The leap from defender to prospector (or the reverse) is beyond most organizations' comfort zones and, therefore, is likely to be resisted. Empirical support for this notion is also found in studies of other industries (Topping and Rudolph, 1989).

Pace of Change. None of the existing health care literature explicitly addresses the rapidity with which strategic changes are initiated and implemented. The shorter time interval studies (Zajac and Shortell, 1989; Shortell, Morrison and Friedman, 1990) suggest that the changes occurred within at least a two-year period as evidenced by both chief executive officers' perceptions and the hospitals' actual market behavior. Some evidence also suggests that organizations staying within their strategic comfort zone had fewer problems in implementing the needed changes and, therefore, were able to do so more quickly than those that did not stay in their comfort zones. At the same time, the content of the new strategy adopted influenced the pace of change. For example, strategies emphasizing an experimental, proactive stance toward the market (for example, the prospector stance) required careful involvement of physicians and ongoing monitoring of the pace of change. At times the implementation processes needed to be accelerated through the formation of task forces and committees. At other times, the process needed to be slowed down as pockets of resistance arose and necessitated regrouping and reeducation tactics.

Duration of Permanence of Change. Once established, how long do new strategies persist? Although the existing studies cover periods of several years, none are of sufficient length to directly address this question. However, 60 percent of those in the national study of system hospitals reported that they planned to continue with present strategies for at least two years (Shortell, Morrison, and Friedman, 1990). (Of the 40 percent who planned to change their strategies, the vast majority intended to become analyzers, again reflecting the strategy makers' beliefs that proactive strategies rather than defensive strategies will better meet evolving environmental demands.) In general, the permanence of an organization's strategy is likely to be a function of the extent to which it continues to help the organization meet and anticipate environmental changes and competitive threats, achieve goals and objectives, and make use of capabilities while remaining consistent with the organization's mission and values. This area requires increased attention.

Effects of Change. On average, little evidence suggests that those who changed their strategies outperformed those who did not in regard to a variety of financial and nonfinancial indicators (Zajac and Shortell, 1989; Shortell, Morrison, and Friedman, 1990). This finding may be due to the relatively short time frame in which performance effects were examined. However, evidence suggests that prospectors and analyzers outperform defenders, particularly in regard to financial indicators and market share. These findings are significant in that they provide empirical support for top management's belief that in the rapidly changing health care environment the analyzer and prospector strategies appear to be the "correct" ones.

The Process of Strategic Adaptation: Building Blocks of a Theory

As shown in Figure 6.2, strategies are a function of the interaction among environments, organizations, managers, markets, and performance. These elements are the building blocks for understanding

Figure 6.2. Elements of a Theory of Strategic Adaptation.

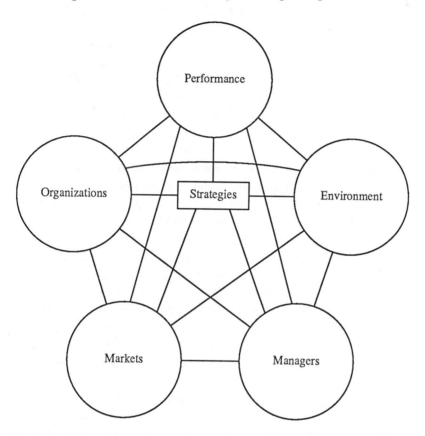

strategy formulation, implementation, and change. Thus, a "theory" of environments, a "theory" of organizations, a "theory" of managerial behavior, a "theory" of markets, and a "theory" of performance are required. Understanding strategic change is an inherently multidisciplinary process in which interdisciplinary research is likely to provide the greatest guidance. The most important elements of each of these building blocks are highlighted and then pulled together into an integrative framework that may be used to guide future research.

Role of Environment. From the perspective of strategic adaptation, the most important characteristic of environments is the nature of change within them—the extent to which change is structural or cyclical in nature (Martell, 1986). Structural changes are relatively permanent qualitative changes in the environment. Cyclical changes are relatively temporary, largely quantitative changes in the environment. The introduction of the Medicare prospective-payment system in 1983 is an example of a structural change in that it resulted in a qualitatively different relationship between hospitals and one of their major payers—the federal government. Faced with condition-specific payment caps, hospitals for the first time had an incentive to provide efficient, less costly care. Examples of cyclical change include a change in the interest rates for financing capital expansion or changes in the rate of inflation in the overall economy. Some periods may be more favorable for expansion of services than others, but the up and down changes are just that—reversible. They may require some adjustment in the organization's behavior but not radical change.

Table 6.1 provides further insight into structural versus cyclical change by summarizing some of the key implications for the strategic-adaptation attributes discussed in the previous section. As shown, structural changes in the environment are likely to have far more important and pervasive implications for strategic adaptation than are cyclical changes. Cyclical changes cannot be ignored but do not require the degree of reorientation or realignment demanded by structural changes.

The distinction between structural and cyclical change applies to both the organization's institutional and its task environment. Some institutional-level changes are structural in nature, such as the increase in the number of women entering the medical profession, while others are cyclical, such as fluctuations in capital markets. Similarly, some changes in the organization's task environment are structural, such as the growth in the out-of-hospital services, while others are cyclical, such as the number of competitors entering or leaving the market. Whether it is dealing with the institutional environment or the task environment, top management's perception of environmental change as structural or cyclical and the implications for the organization are of particular importance.

Role of Managers. It is generally agreed that the organization's top-management team or dominant coalition plays a key role

**Table 6.1. Implications of Structural and Cyclical
Environmental Change for Strategic Adaptation.**

Implications for Strategic Adaptation	Structural	Cyclical
Prevalence	Higher probability of significant and widespread strategic change	Lower probability of significant and widespread strategic change
Direction	In the direction of fitting or matching the perceived requirements of the changed environment in an ongoing fashion	In a direction that can be easily reversed
Magnitude	Substantial; new and different resources and capablities required	Small; minor adjustments in current resources and capabilities required
Pace	As rapid as possible; each day lost cannot be made up	Slow, no overreacting
Duration	Long-term and relatively permanent	Short-term and temporary
Performance Effects	Substantial and long-lasting	Minor and reversible

in both perceiving the need for change and organizing to implement change (Hambrick and Finkelstein, 1987). Success often depends on accurately perceiving the nature of the environmental change as structural or cyclical, understanding the demands that the environmental change places on the organization, and accurately assessing the organization's capabilities to cope with these demands. By misperceiving structural change as cyclical change, managers can underreact to environmental change. In contrast, mistaking cyclical change as structural change can lead to overreaction. For example, hospital executives who thought that Medicare prospective payment (structural change) would be a temporary blip on the screen (cyclical change) made a significant mistake in underreacting and failed to accurately diagnose the qualitatively different implications of this new form of payment. Their hospitals were ill-prepared to deal with the challenges and have largely played catch-up in attempting to cope with the new payment environment. At the same time, other hospital executives overreacted to increases in competition (cyclical change) by offering every diversified service possible; they made the mistake of assuming that every competitor would stay in business and exert long-lasting and permanent influence (structural change).

In general, the perception of the environment as structural or cyclical depends on top management's experience and abilities, the visibility of the change itself, the pervasiveness of the change, and the organization's recent performance. The greater top management's experience and the greater the extent to which top management has been exposed to external events and circumstances and worked outside the current organization, the more likely they are to be able to distinguish between structural and cyclical change. One might also expect that the greater the experience they have had with the organization's core technology and their competitors, the better they will be at perceiving the difference between structural and cyclical change in the task environment.

The more visible the environmental change, the easier it is to detect and to decide whether it is structural or cyclical. For example, a change in the way in which physicians are paid is a highly visible change. In contrast, the changing demographics of a hospital's local community may be less discernible because the change may occur in increments over a period of many years.

The number of groups affected by the change and the importance of these effects (that is, their pervasiveness) also influence management's perception. The greater the degree to which suppliers, customers, and competitors are affected by the environmental change, the greater likelihood that the change will be noticed and perceived as significant by management. For example, many hospitals that initially underestimated the effect of prospective payment eventually saw the impact it was having on other hospitals, major employers, and even suppliers. Recognizing the ripple effect, many hospitals saw the need for significant strategic adaptation and initiated responses that included the joining of systems, consolidation or merger, corporate restructuring, and diversification of services.

Management's recognition of the importance of environmental change will also be influenced by the organization's performance over time and, in particular, in recent years. In general, the more successful the organization has been in the past, the less likely is top management to recognize the need for change. This response may be due less to top management's failure to recognize the importance of the environmental change than to their confidence in the organization's ability to deal with the change with its current strategies. This mind-set is particularly dangerous when the environmental change is structural. Thus, as ironical as it may seem, poor performance in recent years may be a blessing in disguise if it causes top management to reexamine the organization's strategic orientation and ability to deal with the changed environment. In current failure may be sown the seeds of future success.

In addition to accurately assessing the nature of the environmental change, top management must be adept at understanding the demands that the change places on the organization. What are the specific implications for the organization? Simply recognizing prospective payment as an important structural change was not sufficient. It was also necessary to diagnose what it meant for "treating" the organization. For those operating in highly competitive environments, prospective payment might mean the need to develop new services and new revenue streams, and, in turn, to develop new skills and new relationships with physicians. For those operating in a highly regulated environment, it might mean the need to emphasize cost containment and consolidation of staff and services. This response, in turn, might call for considerable education of physicians and nurses and reassurance that the quality of care will not be compromised by cost-cutting efforts. Accurately diagnosing the demands of environmental change is particularly important when the change is structural because of its generally enduring and pervasive nature.

Role of the Organization. As noted, an important top-management responsibility is assessing the capability of the organization to deal with the environmental change. This task involves systematic consideration of the organization's current mission and goals, strategies, design, information-processing abilities, skill mix and experience, and, of course, financial resources. Some hospitals do not change their basic strategic orientation even when they think it is the "correct" thing to do because top management does not believe the organization has the ability to do so (Shortell, Morrison, and Friedman, 1990).

The organization's mission and overall goals provide a starting point for assessment. Has the environment changed so radically that it is beyond the scope of the organization's mission? Does the mission need to be expanded? For example, a hospital that has served the local community for seventy-five years may suddenly need to expand its mission to become a regional health care provider. Conversely, a hospital that has identified itself for years as a regional medical center may need to refocus and downsize its services to a few centers of excellence rather than trying to compete with others across the board.

It is also useful to distinguish between the core and peripheral aspects of the organization's mission. The core comprises the organization's identity—its heart and soul and reason for existence. Typically, this core will not be subject to change even in the face of bankruptcy or closure. In contrast, the peripheral features of the organization's mission are malleable. Not only can they be changed to meet environmental demands, but they often must be in order to protect the organization's core mission.

Existing health care organizational research also suggests that an organization's current strategy is one of the best predictors of whether a switch in strategies will occur. The ability of the organization to deal with the environmental change with its current strategy must be assessed. Among the most important characteristics of the current strategy are its ability to handle complexity, diversity, divisibility, and reversibility (Zaltman, Duncan, and Holbek, 1973; Shortell, Morrison, and Friedman, 1990). If the current strategy can embrace complexity and diversity, then the organization may be able to handle a marked change in its environment. Thus, an analyzer strategy that encompasses the development of new markets and new services (characteristics of a prospector) and that emphasizes efficiency and cost containment (characteristics of a defender) may be complex and diverse enough to deal with a significant environmental change for which it is difficult to predict the ultimate consequences. In this regard, it is of particular interest to note that the most frequently selected strategy in the health care industry has been the analyzer.

The ability of the organization's current strategy to be divided into subcomponents or parts and to be reversed is also important. If the organization's current strategy can be subdivided, it may be able to deal with environmental change without a strategic shift because the ability to subdivide suggests a "loose coupling" (Weick, 1976) of strategic components that permits flexibility in the adaptation process. Similarly, if an organization's current strategy can be undone or retraced to some extent, a major strategic reorientation may be unnecessary. In both cases however, structural environmental change will be a stronger test than will cyclical change. In fact, organizations whose current strategy can be subdivided and reversed should be particularly adept at dealing with cyclical changes in their environments. Precisely for this reason cyclical changes are less likely than structural changes to generate significant strategic shifts.

The organization's current strategy interacts with the organization's design, information-processing practices, and overall skill mix in determining the organization's ability to respond to the changing environment. We refer to the organization's design (functional, divisional, matrix, the level at which decisions are made) its information-processing practices, and its skill mix as the organization's capability. The organization's current strategy and its associated capability combine to determine its strategic comfort zone (Shortell, Morrison, and Friedman, 1990), as previously defined. Making switches to adjacent strategies requires less radical alterations of an organization's current capability and, thus, increases the likelihood of a successful transition. The characteristics of complexity, diversity, divisibility, and reversibility that tend to be associated with different strategies also play a role here. For example, a defender strategy is generally associated with a relatively low degree of complexity and diversity, while a prospector strategy is generally associated with a relatively high degree of complexity and diversity. Once again, structural environmental change rather than cyclical change is likely to place the greater demand on the organization to expand its strategic comfort zone.

The ability of the organization to expand its strategic com-

fort zone will depend largely on its financial resources or its degree
of slack. The greater the available slack, the better the organization's
ability to upgrade its information-processing capabilities, reconfig-
ure its decision-making processes and design, retrain workers, and
purchase new skills. The existence of slack is particularly important
when change is structural. In fact, organizations with little slack
may subconsciously misread or redefine structural environmental
change as cyclical in order to obtain a match with their existing
resources and capabilities. Such redefining is precisely what some
hospitals may have done in the mid-1980s in response to the Medicare prospective-payment system. Also, organizations that have en-
joyed recent financial success without a large capital endowment or
long-standing surplus of slack may accurately diagnose the environmental change as structural but, as previously noted, overesti-
mate their ability to handle the change.

      Role of Markets. Markets are usually treated as part of the
organization's task environment and thus included under the analysis of the environment. But we believe the interaction of organizations and markets to be of sufficient importance to deserve
separate attention. Although many characteristics of markets are
relevant to strategic adaptation, we focus on two of particular importance: entry and exit barriers, and an organization's ability to
create and sustain competitive advantages. Competitive advantage
will be determined largely by the organization's position in the
marketplace relative to current competitors and new competitors
and its ability to exit from markets that are no longer attractive. The
role played by exit barriers is relatively underemphasized in the
literature to date (Porter, 1980).

      In health care, there is almost a bimodal distribution of entry
and exit barriers. On the one hand, entry barriers for the development of new hospitals and high-priced, high-technology services
are relatively high. Such developments usually require considerable
capital, knowledge, and expertise, and often have to meet strict
regulatory requirements. On the other hand, entry barriers for low-
tech services such as health promotion, home health care, and sports
medicine are relatively low, usually requiring little capital and en-
countering few regulatory constraints. Exit barriers for hospitals are

high not only because of their investment in capital and people but also because of their political and social legitimacy. The outcry caused by hospital closures attests to this fact. In contrast, exit barriers for services such as health promotion, home health care, and sports medicine are low because they are less capital intensive and, in some cases, are easily replaced with alternative services.

The key lies in assessing the impact of environmental change (whether structural or cyclical) on the entry and exit barriers for the market in which the organization operates. If the environmental change increases the barriers to entry on the part of other organizations, then there may be less need for a given organization to change its strategies. If the change lowers the barriers to entry, then there may be pressure on the organization to change its strategies in order to respond to the new competitors.

Exit barriers may operate in a more complex fashion than entry barriers. If exit barriers are raised for the firm as a whole, it may be faced with having to make a major strategic reorientation because leaving the business altogether is simply not a viable alternative. If exit barriers are lowered, then dissolution may be a viable strategic alternative. More likely, entry and exit barriers exist for specific units or for product or market segments, and decisions to divest or expand are made at this level. When an exit barrier for a given service is lowered, it may be possible for the organization to divest the service without fundamentally changing its overall strategic orientation.

The most important implication of markets is the ability of the organization to create and sustain a competitive advantage. The challenge is to develop new products and services that meet consumer needs and desires more effectively than those of competitors. Ideally, an organization wants to be the first or at least one of the first to develop a new product or service and then works continuously to erect barriers to prevent others from entering the market. One of the lessons, however, that health care holds for other industries is that the gains that may be achieved from using the "first-mover" strategy (Lieberman and Montgomery, 1988) are short-lived and difficult to sustain without constant differentiation of the product or service. The key lies in developing products and services that are difficult for others to imitate (Barney, 1988) and then to continuously refine or extend the products or services so as to assure their uniqueness in the minds of the consumer.

Role of Performance. It has already been mentioned that the failure to meet performance objectives or poor performance relative to competitors or industry standards is often a trigger for strategic change. However, much of the current literature focuses on traditional financial and accounting indicators of performance such as profit margins, cash flow, and return on equity. Although in the long run these are relevant measures by which the success of many firms' strategies ought to be evaluated, they may not be the most appropriate set of indicators for evaluating short-run strategic effects. Furthermore, they may be too limited to encompass all strategic objectives. Some strategies have short-run objectives, such as preempting a competitor from entering the market or repositioning the organization to deal with future change, that in the short run may be associated with decreased financial performance. In the case of health care organizations, other objectives include improving the quality of services, improving patient care, and meeting the needs of those without the ability to pay for their care. It may be as important to consider the failure to meet these objectives as a cause for initiating strategic change as it is to consider the failure to meet financial goals.

Performance gaps are particularly likely to be triggers for strategic change when the top-management team interprets them as the result of a poor alignment of the organization's current strategy with the nature of the changed environment rather than as the result of a failure in execution or implementation. If a gap is interpreted as a failure in implementation, the tendency will be to redouble the effort or to work smarter but not to change the game plan. Here again, the consequences of misinterpretation are likely to be more serious if the environmental change is structural than if it is cyclical.

Putting the Blocks Together: A Framework
for Further Research

Advances in our understanding of strategic change and adaptation can be made by examining the relationships among the building blocks of environment, organizations, managers, markets, and performance. Central to this examination are the processes of perception, interpretation, and comparison (Ginsberg and Grant, 1985; Dutton and Duncan, 1987; Thomas, 1990). People in organizations, particularly leaders, combine information with their own knowledge and experience in perceiving whether environmental change is structural or cyclical. They also interpret the meaning of the change for their organization, taking into account their internal assessment of the organization's capabilities and their strategic comfort zone and making an external assessment of how the market in which the organization operates—particularly in regard to entry and exit barriers—is influenced by environmental change. They make these interpretations and assessments by comparing the organization's performance with its goals and objectives, stakeholder expectations, and the performance of immediate competitors as well as the industry at large. The overall process is one of comparing the organization's strategic direction with the demands of the environment to arrive at a decision to continue with the current strategic orientation or to adopt a new orientation.

Given our discussion to this point, we can suggest some relationships among the components of the framework in regard to the probability and magnitude of strategic change. These examples are hypotheses to be tested rather than a single integrated theory.

Hypothesis 1: The greater the degree to which environmental change is perceived as structural rather than cyclical, the greater the probability and magnitude of strategic change

Hypothesis 2: The greater the degree to which poor performance is attributed to environmental demands rather than to internal operations, the greater the probability and magnitude of strategic change

Hypothesis 3: The greater the organization's perceived capability of managing a new strategy, the greater the probability and magnitude of strategic change

Hypothesis 4: The greater the degree to which an organization's current strategy lacks characteristics (that is, complexity versus simplicity or diversity versus homogeneity) consistent with environmental demands, the greater the probability and magnitude of strategic change

Hypothesis 5: The greater the extent to which the organization's current strategy is unable to sustain a competitive advantage across an altered set of entry and exit barriers, the greater the probability and magnitude of strategic change

These hypotheses are first-order relationships. In addition, a number of second-order relationships can be suggested involving the factors most likely to be associated with the perceptual, interpretative, and comparative processes that underlie these hypotheses. For example, in regard to the accuracy of perceiving the external environment the following are suggested.

Hypothesis 6: The more varied the skills and experiences of the top-management team, the more accurate their perception of the external environment

Hypothesis 7: The more visible the external change, the more accurate the top-management team's perception of the external environment

Hypothesis 8: The more pervasive the effects of the external environment, the more accurate will be the top-management team's perception of the external environment

Hypothesis 9: The greater the organization's performance gap, the more accurate will be the top-management team's perception of the external environment.

Similarly, in regard to assessing the organization's strategic comfort zone, the following might be suggested:

Hypothesis 10: The more widely shared the organization's mission and goals, the more accurate the assessment of the organization's strategic comfort zone

Hypothesis 11: The greater the understanding of the current strategic orientations requirements in relation to the requirements of alternative strategic orientations, the more accurate the assessment of the strategic comfort zone

Hypothesis 12: The greater the knowledge of current decision practices, information-processing systems, and skill mix, the more accurate the assessment of the organization's strategic comfort zone

Hypothesis 13: The greater the availability of slack resources, the greater the ability to expand the organization's strategic comfort zone.

A number of hypotheses related to performance can also be suggested. These include:

Hypothesis 14: The greater the accuracy of the top-management team's perception of the environment, the better the organization's performance

Hypothesis 15: The greater the degree of match or fit between the organization's capabilities and environmental demands, the better the organization's performance

Hypothesis 16: The greater the degree to which strategic change is undertaken within the organization's strategic comfort zone the better the organization's performance in the long run

A number of interactive hypotheses can also be examined. For example, the relationship between the accuracy of environmental diagnosis and performance is likely to be stronger when change is structural rather than cyclical.

The advantage of the proposed framework is that it integrates a variety of issues and approaches associated with strategic adaptation. It recognizes that adaptation involves the study of relationships and comparative processes. Among the most important of these relationships are those between environmental characteristics and demands and organizational capabilities, between environmental demands and the organization's recent performance and between environmental demands and local market characteristics. In addition, the ability of the top-management team to diagnose accurately the nature of these relationships and interpret their meaning for the organization is important. Thus, strategic adaptation is seen as a dynamic, interactive process between the organization and its environment, a process mediated largely by the organization's leaders. In this regard, one way in which managers can expand their strategic comfort zone and increase organizational capabilities is through participation in interorganizational networks and strategic alliances.

Strategic Alliances

The growth of interorganizational networks and strategic alliances appears to be associated with turbulent environments. In recent years, it has become fashionable to use the term *turbulent* to depict environments of organizations. Originally coined by Emery and Trist (1965) to depict highly complex and rapidly changing environments, turbulence has been somewhat loosely used to describe almost every industry in transition. However, a close inspection of the Emery and Trist definition reveals two general conditions under which the term is appropriate: high interconnectedness of organizations and substantial interdependence between society and the focal organization.

Organizational researchers studying today's turbulent American health care system have tended to neglect studying the interconnectedness and interdependence among organizations and instead have overemphasized amorphous and powerful environmental "forces." We contend that the emphasis on immutable forces, while understandable, may implicitly shape the way that organizational researchers view organization/environment interactions. For example, both the population-ecology and the institutional perspectives in organization theory typically conceive of organizational environments in broad, depersonalized terms as forces that impose either organizational conformity or death. In this vein, Scott and Meyer (1983, p. 149) define an *institutional environment* as "the elaboration of rules and requirements to which individual organizations must conform." It should also be noted that institutional theorists have begun to "move away from a conception of *the* institutional environment to one of multiple institutional environments" (Scott, 1987, p. 498).

We prefer to demystify the discussion of organizational environments by viewing the environment of a health care organization as simply the collection of other specific organizations that are interconnected to or interdependent with it. This health care organization, in turn, is part of the environment for the other organizations. In other words, when a health care organization "looks out" with concern at its turbulent environment, what it sees are other organizations "looking out" at it!

An important implication of this perspective is that the analysis of organization/environment relations shifts away from the question of how an organization fares under the pressures of institutionally demanding or "naturally" selecting environments or both, and moves toward the question of how an organization interacts (for example, competitively or cooperatively) with other relevant, specific organizations. Stated differently, there is value in focusing less on turbulent environments and more on the specific strategic actions of health care organizations that are aimed at confronting—and sometimes contributing to—the overall turbulence in organizational environments. (We do not advocate ignoring relevant environmental issues that are nonorganizational in nature, such as demographic trends. Our view is simply that most relevant environmental forces are, in fact, organizationally created and sustained, and thus are subject to organizational influence.)

However, even here, we suggest that the strategy literature's emphasis on the adaptation efforts of single organizations should be complemented with an increased focus on the strategic-adaptation efforts of the collective set of interdependent organizations (Astley and Fombrun, 1983). The following discussion investigates one such organizational innovation whose growth has coincided with increased environmental turbulence—namely, health care strategic alliances. Formation of these alliances can be viewed as one way in which organizations expand their capabilities and extend their strategic comfort zones.

A health care strategic alliance can be defined as any formal arrangement between two or more health care organizations for purposes of mutual gain. Historically, a variety of multi-institutional arrangements have been found in health care (see DeVries, 1978, or Starkweather, 1971, for basic comparisons of a wide range of such arrangements). However, changes in the health care environment suggest the need to consider additional new forms of alliances as well as to reexamine traditional types of alliances and the motives that drive their formation, growth, and success. Stated differently, we are interested in examining the implications of the forms, functions, and effectiveness of contemporary health care strategic alliances. Before proceeding, however, it is important to discuss the conceptual contributions of the existing health care literature on multi-institutional arrangements.

Previous Views of Multi-Institutional Arrangements. The earliest approaches usually attempted to establish a continuum on which multi-institutional arrangements could be located (Starkweather, 1971; Brown and Lewis, 1976; DeVries, 1978). DeVries (1978, p. 82), for example, arrays multi-dimensional systems on a continuum from "less commitment, more institutional autonomy" to "more commitment, more system control," in the following order: formal affiliation, shared or cooperative services, consortia for planning or education, contract management, lease, corporate ownership but separate management, and complete ownership.

In conceptual terms, Longest (1980) views the growth of multi-institutional systems as the result of an "external dependency relationship" between the hospital and its environment. In doing so, Longest is applying the resource-dependence perspective (put forth by Pfeffer and Salancik, 1978, in the organization-theory literature) to the health care industry. Although Longest uses the term *stabilization strategy* to characterize multihospital arrangements, his view of strategy is somewhat restricted. He states (1980, p. 19): "It is formulated by people for a hospital that exists in relation to an external environment upon which the hospital is highly dependent." When Longest asserts that certain environmental circumstances lead to predictable strategic responses, his deterministic view of hospital actions appears to go even beyond the original notions of Pfeffer and Salancik, although he retreats somewhat from this position in his later work (Longest, 1981).

Fottler, Schermerhorn, Wong, and Money (1982), although also using an "environmental-dependence" approach, do not assume a purely reactive hospital and allow for attempts by hospitals to influence environments. Reviewing the conceptual literature, the authors are rather critical and note that there continue to be limitations to the understanding of interorganizational phenomena. Regarding the state of empirical research on the impact of multi-institutional arrangements, Fottler, Schermerhorn, Wong, and Money (1982, p. 72) view most of the studies as "only semi-empirical, often based on expert testimonies rather than scientific inquiry."

Provan (1984) discusses interorganizational relationships within one type of multihospital system, a consortium. Provan focuses on the single issue of decision-making autonomy, using solely a resource-dependence framework, and acknowledges that he makes "no attempt . . . to relate decision-making autonomy to hospital effectiveness" (p. 498). Despite having limited the scope of the paper, Provan (1984, p. 494) states the interesting view that "although other perspectives are available, they tend to be narrower than resource-dependence as a general framework for understanding interorganizational activity." We suggest that the strategic-management perspective provides a broader and more general framework for understanding interorganizational activity than does the resource-dependence perspective.

D'Aunno and Zuckerman (1987) offer an interesting discussion of how hospital federations may follow a life-cycle model of development. The article, in taking a longitudinal perspective, is an original theoretical contribution to the existing literature on interorganizational arrangements, which has tended to take a static perspective. (Shortell and Zajac, 1988, and Zajac, Golden, and Shortell, 1990, have also attempted to use health care data to examine longitudinal issues in interorganizational arrangements.) One question that arises is whether federations need to progress in the sequence hypothesized by D'Aunno and Zuckerman, or whether managerial actions can substantially alter their evolution. (This question is general to all research that invokes life-cycle models of organizational, product, or industry evolution.)

Luke, Begun, and Pointer (1989) apply Eccles's (1985) notion of the quasi firm to analyze interorganizational arrangements in the health care industry. They also attempt to construct their own "classification of interorganizational relationships" based on two dimensions: tightness of coupling and degree of strategic purpose. The typology is somewhat confusing, however, in that one of their types is the firm, which is not an interorganizational relationship. Another type, called a "latent" firm (an organization that is tightly coupled but has a low degree of strategic purpose), is also not an interorganizational relationship. In addition, the examples given for a latent firm include organizations such as large public utilities whose top managers would probably take exception to having their organizations characterized as not having a high strategic purpose. Another difficulty is that Luke, Begun, and Pointer equate permanence with degree of importance. This need not always be the case.

To summarize, the prominent feature of most of the existing literature has been the development of typological approaches, similar to those offered by Starkweather (1971), Brown and Lewis

(1976), and DeVries (1978). These typologies have been useful in documenting and describing the common and different features of a wide range of interorganizational arrangements in health care. Researchers now need to explore the significance of these commonalities and differences. For example, what differences should an organization expect if it were to choose one form rather than another? We argue that the existing health care—and general organization-theory—literature has not yet developed an adequate response to this question. We further argue, however, that there may not be a clear-cut answer, and that the question itself may be misleading. More specifically, we believe that several of the forms of conventional wisdom about strategic alliances should be challenged.

Myths About Multi-Institutional Arrangements. As noted, DeVries (1978) and others have arrayed multi-institutional systems on a continuum of autonomy to control. Almost without exception, however, these rank orderings reflect the degree of ownership, with complete ownership being equated with the highest form of control. We argue that to equate ownership with control can often be misleading, and we use a simple, publicly visible example from a non-health care setting to demonstrate our point.

Myth #1: Degree of ownership equals degree of control. It is well known that McDonald's Corporation is interested in maintaining control over its raw materials to ensure that quality is highly consistent. In dealing with its suppliers, one might therefore expect that McDonald's would prefer an interorganizational arrangement that would involve ownership of suppliers in order to have substantial control. This is not the case however. With no ownership interests, McDonald's simply communicates its quality requirements to the supplier organizations, and the organizations are quick to oblige.

How can this be? Two factors seem to be relevant. The first is obvious: McDonald's, by virtue of its size, enjoys substantial relative power in its relationship with suppliers (McDonald's represents a large portion of any food supplier's business). Having this power obviates, in large part, the need for McDonald's also to own some or all of its suppliers' assets. Ownership and control are essentially separated in this case. The second reason involves the establishment of a tradition of mutual gain and cooperation. Specifically, McDonald's has made it a policy to be loyal to high-quality suppliers and to use its size to protect suppliers from dramatic swings in sales revenue. In this way, both parties have incentives to ensure a long-term cooperative relationship with no ownership interests. Some parallel is apparent in the relationships that currently exist between hospitals and physicians.

This simplified example is not intended to show that ownership and control are usually uncorrelated. Rather, it demonstrates that tight control can exist even when there is no ownership. In other words, the theoretical continuum that is popularly used for locating different types of health care strategic alliances may be in need of reevaluation.

This reevaluation of the forms of strategic alliances brings us to a second popular misconception.

Myth #2: Form equals function. Researchers, by focusing on the different types or forms of health care strategic alliances, have implicitly assumed that certain forms imply certain functions and even certain outcomes. If a single form could serve multiple functions, researchers would have no interest in discussing the differences among forms. Zajac (1986) addresses this issue, in part, in his analysis of contract-management arrangements. He argues that organizations choosing to engage in a similar type of strategic alliance may have widely varying intentions and that expected performance will vary correspondingly. He thereby suggests that it may not be reasonable to expect a particular form of interorganizational arrangement to translate into a particular performance result. And, in fact, Zajac found that the performance outcomes of similar contract-management arrangements differed depending on the strategic intentions or orientations of the organizations involved.

This finding suggests a general neglect of the concept of strategic orientation in previous research on interorganizational arrangements. The form of alliance used may be much less important in suggesting particular performance outcomes than the strategic intentions, as articulated by key decision makers, that motivate that choice of alliance. In other words, the form of the alliance is not a good predictor of what the alliance can achieve. Outcomes will also be influenced by key decision makers' perceptions of environmental change as being cyclical or structural. The implication of this line of argument is that it is important for researchers to consider the strategic intentions of participant organizations when deciding which performance outcome(s) to include in their analysis of health care strategic alliances.

The issue of performance arises in the third misconception about strategic alliances.

Myth #3: Strategic alliances are inherently risky. Some researchers have argued that strategic alliances, by their very nature, are risky endeavors (Harrigan, 1985). From this perspective, the cooperative links between two or more organizations are viewed as somewhat fragile, exposing each party to the risk that the other party or parties may not continue to cooperate as expected. Luke, Begun, and Pointer (1989) also characterize their quasi firms as inherently unstable. And the business press has had a penchant for describing, in detail, particular joint ventures or other alliances that failed (for example, one of us was recently approached by a reporter who wanted to do a story on the five biggest joint-venture failures).

We argue that this fixation on riskiness may be misguided. Specifically, we contend that any assessment of the risk of strategic alliances should be balanced with an assessment of the expected returns of the alliance in financial performance, political influence, innovation, and organizational learning, and an assessment of the opportunity cost of not engaging in a strategic alliance. Regarding the expected returns, although financial performance is an obvious outcome to consider when analyzing the success or failure of a strategic alliance, it is not clear that it should be considered the most important outcome. For example, innovation may be a driving force behind strategic alliances (Zajac, Golden, and Shortell, 1990), and, more generally, alliances may be viewed as a desirable way for organizations to learn about new markets, services, and ways of doing business. These outcomes may be negatively correlated with financial performance, at least in the short run (Shortell and Zajac, 1988).

Regarding opportunity cost, the baseline for comparison when considering a joint venture is not Is it risky?, but What is riskiest: going it alone, doing nothing, or engaging in an alliance?

What is likely to expand the organization's capabilities and strategic comfort zone? Riskiness is not necessarily a problem per se. For example, the virtues of entrepreneurship are often extolled, despite the high risk involved. Strategic alliances may appear risky when the baseline comparison is not made explicit, but when compared with attempting a de novo entry into a new market or ignoring the market altogether, entering an alliance may seem like a relatively low-risk proposition.

Advantages of a Strategic-Management Perspective. We would contend that the debatable logic underlying these three myths becomes obvious when one takes a strategic-management perspective. Perhaps a historical overemphasis on the structural features of strategic alliances is responsible for each of the three myths. In any event, gaining an understanding of the strategic objectives driving such cooperative activities is the first and most important step toward understanding the effectiveness of strategic alliances.

We hope that our discussion of strategic alliances and strategic adaptation in general has demonstrated the advantages of complementing population-ecology and institutional-theory perspectives with a strategic-management perspective. In this regard, we would like to end our discussion on a provocative note by making an observation and posing a question. When we look at health care, we see flourishing new organizational and interorganizational forms and activities. Which theory seems best suited for explaining these developments: the standard population-ecology approach, which, as Astley (1985) notes, is limited to observing selection and retention (rather than variation) in a given population of organizations over time; the institutional approach, which stresses the conformity and homogeneity of organizations (DiMaggio and Powell, 1983); or the strategic-management approach, which emphasizes organizational adaptation and change? We hope that this chapter, and other chapters in this book, will stimulate further discussion of this issue.

References

Alexander, J. A., Morlock, L. L., and Gifford, B. D. "The Effects of Corporate Restructuring on Hospital Policymaking." *Health Services Research*, 1988, *23*, 311–337.

Andrews, K. R. *The Concept of Corporate Strategy.* Homewood, Ill.: Dow Jones—Irwin, 1971.

Ansoff, H. I. *Corporate Strategy: An Analytic Approach to Business Policy for Growth and Expansion.* New York: McGraw-Hill, 1965.

Ansoff, H. I. "Strategic Management of Technology." *Journal of Business Strategy,* 1987, *7,* 28–39.

Astley, W. G. "The Two Ecologies: Population and Community Perspectives on Organizational Evolution." *Administrative Science Quarterly,* 1985, *30,* 224–242.

Astley, W. G., and Fombrun, C. J. "Collective Strategy: Social Ecology of Organizational Environments." *Academy of Management Review,* 1983, *8,* 576–587.

Barney, J. B. *The Context of Formal Strategic Planning and the Economic Performance of Firms.* Strategy Group Working Paper Series 88-005. College Station: Department of Management, Texas A&M University, 1988.

Brown, M., and Lewis, H. L. *Hospital Management Systems: Multi-Unit Organizations and Delivery of Health Care.* Germantown, Md.: Aspen Systems Corp., 1976.

Burgelman, R. A. *The Intra-Organizational Ecology of Strategy Making and Organizational Adaptation: A Conceptual Integration.* Stanford, Calif.: Strategic Management Program, Graduate School of Business, Stanford University, 1987.

Chandler, A. D., Jr. *Strategy and Structure: Chapters in the History of the Industrial Enterprise.* Cambridge, Mass.: MIT Press, 1962.

Clement, J. P. "Does Hospital Diversification Improve Financial Outcomes?" *Medical Care,* 1987, *25,* 988–1001.

D'Aunno, T. A., and Zuckerman, H. S. "A Life Cycle Model of Organizational Federations: The Case of Hospitals." *Academy of Management Review,* 1987, *12,* 534–545.

DeVries, R. A. "Strength in Numbers." *Journal of the American Hospital Association,* 1978, *55,* 81–84.

DiMaggio, P. J., and Powell, W. W. "The Iron Cage Revisited: Institutional Isomorphism and Collective Rationality in Organizational Fields." *American Sociological Review,* 1983, *48,* 147–160.

Dutton, J. E., and Duncan, R. B. "The Creation of Momentum for

Change Through the Process of Strategic Issue Diagnosis." *Strategic Management Journal*, 1987, *8*, 279–295.

Eccles, R. G. *The Transfer Pricing Problem: A Theory for Practice.* Lexington, Mass.: Lexington Books, 1985.

Emery, F. E., and Trist, E. L. "The Causal Texture of Organizational Environments." *Human Relations*, 1965, *18*, 21–32.

Fahey, L., and Christensen, H. "Evaluating the Research on Strategy Content." *Journal of Management*, 1986, *12* (2), 167–183.

Fottler, M. D., Schermerhorn, J., Wong, J., and Money, W. H. "Multi-Institutional Arrangements in Health Care: Review, Analysis, and a Proposal for Future Research." *Academy of Management Review*, 1982, *7*, 67–79.

Ginn, G. O. "Strategic Adaptation in the Hospital Industry." *Health Services Research*, forthcoming.

Ginsberg, A., and Grant, J. H. "Research on Strategic Change: Theoretical and Methodological Issues." *Proceedings of the Academy of Management*, Aug. 1985.

Hambrick, D. C., and Finkelstein, S. "Managerial Discretion: A Bridge Between Polar Views and Organizational Outcomes." In B. Staw and L. L. Cummings (eds.), *Research in Organizational Behavior.* Vol. 7. Greenwich, Conn.: JAI, 1987.

Hannan, M. T., and Freeman, J. "Structural Inertia and Organizational Change." *American Sociological Review*, 1984, *49*, 149–164.

Harrigan, K. R. *Managing for Joint Venture Success.* Lexington, Mass.: Lexington Books, 1985.

Huff, A. S. and Reger, R. K. "A Review of Strategic Process Research." *Journal of Management*, 1987, *13* (2), 211–236.

Keats, B. W., Conant, J. S., and Mokwa, M. P., "Strategic Orientation and Relative Effectiveness Among Health Maintenance Organizations." Paper presented at meeting of the Academy of Management, Anaheim, Calif., Aug. 1988.

Kimberly, J. R., and Zajac, E. J. "Strategic Adaptation in Health Care Organizations: Implications for Theory and Research." *Medical Care Review*, 1985, *42* (2), 267–302.

Lieberman, M. B., and Montgomery, D. B. "First-Mover Advantages." *Strategic Management Journal*, 1988, *9*, 41–58.

Longest, B. B. "A Conceptual Framework for Understanding the

Multihospital Arrangement Strategy." *Health Care Management Review*, 1980, *5*, 17-24.

Longest, B. B. "An External Dependence Perspective of Organizational Strategy and Structure: A Community Hospital Case." *Hospital and Health Services Administration*, Spring 1981, pp. 50-69.

Luke, R. D., and Begun, J. W. "Strategic Orientations of Small Multihospital Systems." *Health Services Research*, 1988, *23* (5), 597-618.

Luke, R. D. Begun, J. W., and Pointer, D. D. "Quasi Firms: Strategic Interorganizational Forms in the Health Care Industry." *Academy of Management Review*, 1989, *14* (1), 9-19.

Martell, L. *Mastering Change*. New York: Mentor, 1986.

Mick, S. S., and Conrad, D. A. "The Decision to Integrate Vertically in Health Care Organizations." *Journal of Hospital and Health Services Administration*, 1988, *33*, 345-360.

Miles, R. E., and Snow, C. C. *Organizational Strategy, Structure, and Process*. New York: McGraw-Hill, 1978.

Peters, J. P., and Tseng, S. *Managing Strategic Change in Hospitals: Ten Success Stories*. Chicago: American Hospital Association, 1983.

Pfeffer, J., and Salancik, G. R. *The External Control of Organizations: A Resource Dependence Perspective*. New York: Harper & Row, 1978.

Porter, M. E. *Competitive Strategy: Techniques for Analyzing Industries and Competitors*. New York: Free Press, 1980.

Porter, M. E. *Competitive Advantage: Creating and Sustaining Superior Performance*. New York: Free Press, 1985.

Provan, K. G. "Interorganizational Cooperation and Decision Making Autonomy in a Consortium Multihospital System." *Academy of Management Review*, 1984, *9*, 494-504.

Schendel, D. E., and Hofer, C. W. *Strategic Management: A New View of Business Policy and Planning*. Boston: Little, Brown, 1979.

Scott, W. R. *Organizations: Rational, Natural, and Open Systems*. (2nd ed.) Englewood Cliffs, N.J.: Prentice-Hall, 1987.

Scott, W. R., and Meyer, J. W. "The Organization of Societal Sectors." In J. W. Meyer and W. R. Scott (eds.), *Organizational*

Environments: Ritual and Rationality. Beverly Hills, Calif.: Sage, 1983.

Shortell, S. M., Morrison, E. M., and Friedman, B. *Strategic Choices for America's Hospitals: Managing Change in Turbulent Times.* San Francisco: Jossey-Bass, 1990.

Shortell, S. M., Morrison, E. M., and Hughes, S. L. "The Keys to Successful Diversification. Lessons from Leading Hospital Systems." *Hospital and Health Services Administration,* 1989, *34,* 471–492.

Shortell, S. M., Morrison, E. M., and Robbins, S. "Strategy Making in Health Care Organizations: A Framework and Agenda for Research." *Medical Care Review,* 1985, *42,* 219–265.

Shortell, S. M., Wickizer, T., and Wheeler, J. *Hospital-Physician Joint Ventures: Results from a National Demonstration in Primary Care.* Ann Arbor, Mich.: Health Administration Press, 1984.

Shortell, S. M., and Zajac, E. J. "Internal Corporate Joint Ventures: Development Processes and Performance Outcomes." *Strategic Management Journal,* 1988, *9,* 527–542.

Starkweather, D. B. "Health Facility Mergers: Some Conceptualizations." *Medical Care,* 1971, *9,* 468–478.

Thomas, J. B. "Hospitals as Interpretation Systems: The Role of Top Management Information Processing Structure and Strategy Type." *Health Services Research,* forthcoming.

Topping, S., and Rudolph, P. M. "Strategic Adaptation and Changes: Positions and Patterns in One Industry." Paper presented at the meeting of the Business Policy and Planning Division, Academy of Management, Washington, D.C., Aug. 1989.

Weick, K. E. "Educational Organizations as Loosely Coupled Systems." *Administrative Science Quarterly,* 1976, *21,*1–19.

Williamson, O. E. *Markets and Hierarchies: Analysis and Antitrust Implications.* New York: Free Press, 1975.

Zajac, E. J. "Organizations, Environments, and Performance: A Study of Contract Management in Hospitals." Unpublished doctoral dissertation, University of Pennsylvania, 1986.

Zajac, E. J., Golden, B. R., and Shortell, S. M. "New Organizational Forms for Enhancing Innovation: The Case of Internal Corporate Joint Ventures." *Management Science,* forthcoming.

Zajac, E. J., and Shortell, S. M. "Changing Generic Strategies: Likelihood, Direction and Performance Implications." *Strategic Management Journal*, 1989, *10*, 413–430.

Zaltman, G., Duncan, R., and Holbek, J. *Innovations and Organizations*. New York: Wiley, 1973.

7

Technology Diffusion and Ecological Analysis: The Case of Magnetic Resonance Imaging

Laura Roper Renshaw
John R. Kimberly
J. Sanford Schwartz

Sophisticated new technologies are being developed and used in the diagnosis and treatment of illness with increasing frequency. Costs associated with the development of these new technologies are high. Benefits are not always obvious. Thus, providers have a substantial interest in developing policies to either slow or accelerate the pace of diffusion. Development of such policies, however, presumes an understanding of the many factors that influence technology adoption.

Studies of the process of the adoption of medical innovations (for example, Coleman, Katz, and Menzel, 1966; Greer, 1984) typically have employed standard diffusion models to describe and explain observed patterns. As the reality these models are trying to capture has become increasingly complex, however, the limitations

Note: Work on this chapter was funded in part by the National Center for Health Services Research and Health Care Technology, Grant #5RO1 HS 05424. We also wish to thank Alan Hillman and Mark Pauly of the University of Pennsylvania and Michel Berry, director of the Centre de Recherche en Gestion, Ecole Polytechnique, Paris, France, for their advice, support, and encouragement.

of these models have become evident. The Medicare Prospective Payment System (PPS), in particular, has changed the context in which medical diffusion takes place by altering the incentives for efficient production of services. In addition, in response to new opportunities, new actors are entering the health care marketplace, increasing both competition and uncertainty. More significantly, perhaps, the hospital is no longer the sole, or sometimes even the primary, adopter of costly medical technology. Other entities such as physician groups, freestanding centers, and provider networks have been formed to deliver medical services and often to invest in new technologies. Thus, a variety of organizations within communities and local market areas are adopting medical technologies. New perspectives are required to capture the new complexities.

We have been examining the rate and pattern of diffusion of magnetic resonance imaging (MRI) in the early and mid-1980s. In so doing, we have found it useful to supplement traditional diffusion theory with concepts from organizational ecology to help explain observed patterns. Our basic argument is that although environmental factors, such as the imposition of PPS, constrained hospitals' adoption of the technology in the short term, they also created opportunities for other providers—specifically, physician groups and venture-capital firms—to enter the market for high-technology services. This competition, in turn, stimulated reactions from hospitals, which engaged in a range of innovative ways of financing, acquiring, and ensuring access to these technologies. This dynamic altered the expected extent and patterns of technological innovation.

Organizational ecology argues that environmental variables are the primary determinants of organizational entry, transformation, and failure; those organizations survive that best "fit" environmental conditions. An organization's ability to respond adaptively to change, however, is limited by the inertia built into its structures and procedures (Hannan and Freeman, 1977; Hannan and Freeman, 1984) and by what Simon (1957) refers to as bounded rationality—that is, limitations on managers' abilities to understand a complex environment. Thus, we might expect to see considerable volatility in populations of organizations, particularly those confronting rapidly changing environments where considerable adaptability is required to survive (conditions that existed in the health care environment in the 1980s). Ecological analysis is most certainly limited in its ability to explain the diffusion patterns of innovations in medical technology; however, we argue that components of the approach can, in conjunction with standard diffusion theory, lead to an increased appreciation of the dynamic nature of technology diffusion in health care under new and turbulent environmental conditions.

Context and Pattern of MRI Diffusion

MRI is a diagnostic technology that makes electronic images of the head and body using a combination of a highly powerful magnet, radiofrequency pulses, and computers. It is an expensive technology to buy and maintain. Purchasing and siting an MRI unit costs $1 to $2 million, depending on the type and size of the unit and the need for construction of special structures to support the weight of the magnet and to offer protection from the effects of the magnetism generated when the equipment is in use. Furthermore, routine maintenance costs average $100,000 a year (Evens, Jost, and Evens, 1985; Evens and Evens, 1988). The technology first became available for clinical use in December 1981.

In 1983 a new system was established for paying hospitals for the inpatient care provided to Medicare beneficiaries. PPS paid hospitals a fixed fee, assigned at the time of discharge, for each Medicare inpatient, based on the Diagnosis Related Group (DRG) to which the patient belonged on entry into the hospital. Under PPS, if the cost of the patient's stay exceeds the payment to the hospital for that patient's DRG assignment, the hospital loses money. If the patient can be cared for safely at lower cost than the government's payment, the hospital makes money. The overall purpose of PPS is to create a financial incentive for hospitals to provide efficient care for Medicare inpatients, in part through improved management of resources and in part through the elimination of unnecessary practices and overly long hospital stays. PPS increases competition among providers because a hospital can spread its high fixed costs among more patients if it increases its market share—by the number of people admitted for inpatient care. Under PPS hospitals assume increased financial risk for technology purchases and utilization. Thus, it was hoped that PPS would lead to more "rational" technology adoption as hospitals more carefully assessed the clinical value and financial impact of existing and new services (U.S. Congress, 1983; Anderson and Steinberg, 1984). Under PPS it was expected that the rate of technology adoption by hospitals would slow. The impact of PPS was reinforced by the adoption of similar policies by many private insurers.

Some analysts predicted that these policies would not necessarily slow the rate of diffusion overall; rather they would cause hospitals to shift provision of such services to outpatient settings, where they were still reimbursed on a fee-for-service basis (Davis, Andersen, and Steinberg, 1984). Such predictions have been largely borne out in the case of MRI. The rate of diffusion far outpaced the predictions of industry insiders. By the end of 1987 there were over 550 operational units. However, in contrast to past experience with other imaging technologies (for example, computed-tomography scanners), for which hospitals were the principal purchasers, less than half of all MRI units operating at the end of 1986 were fully owned by hospitals. Aside from the traditional form of hospital ownership of expensive, sophisticated medical technology, there were four other common ownership arrangements: joint hospital/ physician-group ownership; full ownership by a physician or physician group; ownership by venture capitalists or some form of intermediary organization (that is, any organization, excluding MRI manufacturing companies and their subsidiaries, that facilitates acquisition of MRI units by providing a range of services such as consulting, financing, management, or leasing through the establishment of contractual relationships with hospitals or physician groups); ownership by a hospital consortium, sometimes also including one or more physician groups.

In the first two years of its availability, hospitals were the main purchasers of MRI. Beginning in 1985 and particularly in 1986, however, freestanding imaging organizations, most frequently owned by physician groups, rapidly entered the MRI market (Hillman and Schwartz, 1985, 1986). Beginning in 1986 and more dramatically in 1987, purchase patterns shifted back to hospitals, although often with nontraditional ownership arrangements such as joint ventures with medical staff and various types of leases. Indeed, approximately 25 percent of the units that became operational in 1986 were leased (Schwartz and others, 1988).

These overall national trends, however, mask considerable local and regional variation in the rate and extent of diffusion, siting, and ownership arrangements. Some local markets have traditional, hospital-dominated, ownership patterns. Other markets are characterized almost exclusively by freestanding sites, while still other markets have mixed ownership patterns. Some markets have been heavily penetrated by intermediary groups, while others have not. Finally, leasing is popular in some markets and not in others. The interesting question for the student of diffusion theory, then, is not only what accounts for different rates of diffusion but also what accounts for the patterns of diffusion in different markets. Our objective is to develop a theoretical perspective that both embraces and helps to account for this variety.

Strengths and Limitations of Diffusion Theory

Traditional diffusion theory has concentrated almost exclusively on analyzing the factors that distinguish adopters of innovations from nonadopters and determining the factors that explain different rates of diffusion in different communities or markets. Rogers (1983), in his thorough review of the diffusion literature, contends that there is widespread consensus about the three main elements of the diffusion model: the technology itself, characteristics of potential adopters, and the environment.

The technology itself has a number of characteristics that affect the rapidity of the technology's diffusion. These characteristics include advantages relative to existing technologies, compatibility with the knowledge and skills of potential users, complexity, ease of testing and of assessing the results (trialability), and observability of advantages.

Potential adopters, be they individuals or organizations, are characterized by traits that make them more or less likely to adopt an innovation. Important individual characteristics that influence the likelihood and speed of adoption of innovations include cosmopolitan orientation, socioeconomic status, education, and links with communication channels and change agents. Among the important organizational characteristics that affect the likelihood and speed of technology adoption are centralization, complexity, formalization, degree of organizational slack, and organizational integration.

The environmental characteristics of significance tend to be case specific and often differ across social science disciplines. In general, technology-diffusion models deal with such factors as system norms, communication patterns, and various sociological and economic factors. In empirical research, the environment is often treated as being static, even though diffusion theory emphasizes the dynamic nature of the process. Cross-sectional studies are common. When efforts are made to incorporate change, they are often limited (for example, studies of the percentage change in per capita income over a designated time period).

The model, then, consists of one set of principal actors—the potential adopters—who are, in effect, exposed to the innovation and to environmental influences, and who eventually make a decision to adopt or not to adopt. The model, at least conceptually, is dynamic in that early adoptions affect subsequent adoption decisions. The appeal of the model is its simplicity, its generality, and its broad applicability.

Most diffusion studies in the health sector have focused on determining the factors associated with hospital adoption of technology. Studies have considered such hospital characteristics as size, location, number of specialists, teaching status, degree of decentralization, and research orientation (Cromwell, Ginsburg, Hamilton, and Sumner, 1975; Cromwell and Kanak, 1982; Greer and Zakhar, 1979; National Research Council and Institute of Medicine, 1979; Kimberly and Evanisko, 1981; Kaluzny, Veney, and Gentry, 1974; Rapoport, 1978; Romeo, Wagner, and Lee, 1984; Russell, 1979; Sloan, Valvona, and Perrin, 1986). Other organizational characteristics studied include decision-making structure, power sharing, interest-group interactions and medical-staff sophistication and training (Greer, 1977; Kimberly and Evanisko, 1981; National Research Council and Institute of Medicine, 1979). Compared with the rather consistent findings about the characteristics of individuals who are early adopters of innovations (Andersen and Jay, 1985;

Becker, 1970; Becker, Sarel, and Gardner, 1985; Coleman, Katz, and Menzel, 1966; Frost, 1985; Kimberly, 1978), the organizational characteristics associated with early adoption are much less clear. The organizational factors that tend to be positively associated with technology adoption are large size (in virtually every study), the existence of hospital teaching and research activities, hospital ownership of the technology, and urban location. Decentralization of hospital resource allocation and medical-staff sophistication and training have some importance (Greer, 1977; Kimberly and Evanisko, 1981; National Research Council and Institute of Medicine, 1979), although the size of the institution consistently has the most explanatory power.

Diffusion models incorporate a number of environmental variables. These variables include measures of demand, competition, and regulation. Demand variables include population size and population growth rate, extent of physician and specialist concentration in market areas, percentage of the population eligible for Medicare, and per capita income. The competition variables are not well developed, but include measures of market share like the Herfindahl index and the four-hospital concentration ratio, as well as enrollment per capita in health maintenance organizations (HMOs). Regulatory variables considered include the presence and stringency of certificate-of-need (CON) and rate regulations. Findings on the impact of environmental variables on diffusion of innovations among hospitals have been inconsistent, varying with the technologies studied (Cromwell and Kanak, 1982; Romeo, Wagner, and Lee, 1984; Russell, 1979; Sloan, Valvona, and Perrin, 1986). The lack of consistent findings is partly attributable to inadequate measures in the case of competition and to lack of data on both competition and third-party payment (Russell, 1979; Sloan, Valvona, and Perrin, 1986).

The traditional diffusion model is not without problems. Three limitations are particularly noteworthy. First, and somewhat paradoxically, the theory appears to assume a relatively stable set of environmental conditions as the context for diffusion. Recent developments in the health sector, particularly the imposition of PPS, suggest turbulence rather than stability and highlight the importance of environmental variables in the explanation of organizational outcomes. The consequences of environmental volatility may overwhelm structural and managerial variations. An adequate theoretical perspective must be sensitive to volatility, as well as to stability, in environmental conditions.

A second limitation is that diffusion theory focuses exclusively on adoption by existing organizations. One of the most interesting aspects of MRI diffusion has been that new organizations have been formed for the purpose of owning and operating the technology (Kimberly and others, 1989, 1990). An adequate theoretical perspective cannot overlook this important phenomenon.

Third, diffusion research typically considers a restricted number of actors. Generally the hospital or the population of hospitals in a market area is the unit of analysis, and no other organization is found in the explanatory equation except insofar as competition variables are included. Yet, in the case of MRI, several different types of organizations are adopting the technology and others are actively promoting its diffusion. An adequate theoretical perspective must be attuned to the significance of organizational contexts.

Organizational Ecology

How might thinking in ecological terms usefully supplement standard diffusion theory? In our view, ecological approaches have particular relevance for the analysis of the diffusion of MRI under changed environmental conditions. In the rapidly developing domain of organizational ecology, three questions tend to underlie empirical research: What accounts for the founding of organizations? What accounts for the failure of organizations? What accounts for the transformation of organizations?

These questions can be approached in several ways. One approach takes the organization as the unit of analysis and some measure of performance (usually survival) as the independent variable. In this approach, factors such as the age and size of the organization or generalist-versus-specialist strategies are the parameters that determine the organization's ability to adapt (Alexander, Kaluzny, and

Middleton, 1986; Brittain and Freeman, 1980; Carroll, 1984; Marple, 1982).

A second approach treats the environment as the unit of analysis, and entry, exit, or transformation of organizations as the independent variable. The empirical work adopting this approach has dealt with organizational founding and entrepreneurship at either the national or community level (Aldrich and Stern, 1983; Delacroix and Carroll, 1983; Pennings, 1982).

The third approach, referred to as community or population demographics, treats competing organizations as the unit of analysis and population growth rates as the dependent variable (Astley and Fombrun, 1984). The major concern is how competitive intensity within a given community affects organizational entry, exit, and strategy. The two principal strategies considered have been opportunistic (in which organizations attempt to be the first to exploit perceived opportunities) and competitive (in which organizations emphasize efficiency and price competition) (Brittain and Wholey, 1986). This approach is the least developed but holds considerable promise for sophisticated analysis of the relationships among organizational behavior, environmental conditions, and survival and transformation rates.

As best we can tell, ecological analysis has not been specifically applied to the diffusion of innovations in medical technology. As noted, a distinguishing characteristic of the diffusion of MRI has been the formation of organizations for the specific purpose of owning and operating the technology. In addition, we found that except for size and teaching status, hospital structural and managerial characteristics (such as the composition of the board of trustees and the formal decision-making process) influenced the timing of adoption and the nature of the financial arrangements far less than strategic initiatives taken in anticipation of, or in reaction to, the self-interested actions of the hospital's own radiology staff or the initiatives of other hospitals in the market area, or both (Kimberly and others, 1989). The longitudinal character of ecological approaches and the emphasis on environmental conditions and patterns of entry and exit are well suited to address-

ing many of the issues raised by our observations about the diffusion of MRI.

Environmental Factors

When we shift from an organizational to a community focus, the
question of interest becomes whether common patterns of ownership and density of units characterize similar market areas over the
long term. To what extent does the principle of isomorphism operate—that is, to what extent do similar conditions create similar
organizational configurations?

The diffusion of MRI is strongly influenced by the environment in which potential adopters make their investment decisions.
Judging from our research (Kimberly and others, 1989), three of the
most important environmental characteristics that shape the investment decision are environmental munificence, environmental uncertainty, and competition. The three characteristics are interrelated
but conceptually distinct. It is useful to think of the environment
in such multilevel, multidimensional terms to avoid overlooking
important influences (Betton and Dess, 1985, p. 754; Ulrich, 1987,
p. 143; Young, 1988, passim). Any health care organization operates
in the context of community, state, and national economic, political, and social trends. Some of these factors are more decisive than
others in shaping the diffusion process and in influencing the long-
term survival of MRI units, although the factors may not be those
anticipated by policy makers or perceived by managers. The analytical challenge is to disaggregate the environment and identify those
components that are particularly significant.

Despite economic constraints faced by hospitals, the resource
environment was, in many respects, favorable to medical-
technology diffusion in the early and mid-1980s, in large part because changes in the environment stimulated competition. On the
one hand, nonhospital actors (such as physician groups, outpatient
clincs, and intermediary organizations), who were not directly confronted with many of the resource and regulatory constraints imposed on hospitals, were able to take advantage of opportunities
presented by a rapidly changing and uncertain health care environment. On the other hand, hospitals, despite confronting economic

constraints introduced by PPS, responded to competitive pressures from both hospital and nonhospital providers by seeking innovative ways to acquire technology at reduced financial risk to themselves. The evolving pattern of diffusion reflects, in aggregate, trade-offs made by individual hospitals among access to the technology, control over its use, and risks associated with that type of investment.

Environmental munificence can be defined as the supply of available resources required for organizational survival. At the time hospitals became interested in the clinical potential of MRI, the health care environment was becoming increasing economically restrictive. The government had cut back Medicare payments, physicians' fees, and Medicaid block grants, while private insurers increasingly were not willing to pay for procedures that did not meet strict criteria of medical necessity. Yet to characterize the environment as resource poor is inaccurate. At least initially after the imposition of PPS, hospitals by and large showed record profits (Feder, Hadley, and Zuckerman, 1987), and physicians' real earnings increased significantly (although the American Medical Association attributed this increase to longer working hours). However, many saw these initial profits as temporary. Hospital administrators were beginning to evaluate services at least partly on the basis of their income-earning potential as they anticipated the onset of less generous reimbursement.

In contrast to the health care environment, the overall economic environment was unequivocally expansionary, at least until the October 1987 stock-market crash. In this environment entrepreneurship was encouraged and much capital and many investors were available for new ventures. Physicians, some of whom were beginning to feel the pinch on their incomes from Medicare-payment freezes, high malpractice-insurance rates, and declines in the number of fee-for-service patients, were looking for additional sources of income and were among the potential investors.

The diffusion literature repeatedly has indicated that specialists are the initiators of technology-adoption efforts (Coleman, Katz, and Menzel, 1966). Yet under PPS specialists found that their traditional means of access to new technology, their hospital, often was unwilling to make sizable investments under conditions of considerable uncertainty. These conditions created an opportunity for physicians to take advantage of the potential demand for MRI (to exploit a market niche), especially in states where CON legislation regulated technology adoption by hospitals but did not regulate technology adoption by nonhospital providers.

Environmental munificence can also be defined by the demand for a service or product—that is, the degree to which the environment can support new growth. The rate and extent of the diffusion of a new technology obviously are functions of the level of demand. However, medical technologies are somewhat distinct from nonmedical technologies (videocassette recorders, personal computers) for two reasons. First, many medical technologies have a virtually guaranteed initial market—the large teaching hospitals that frequently enter into agreements with manufacturers to conduct research and refine clinical applications in exchange for subsidization of the technology or that feel the need to have access to and gain early experience with innovative technologies. Second, the adopters of medical technology, unlike adopters of consumer goods, have a vested interest in promoting its use. Specialists (in the case of MRI, radiologists, and, to a lesser degree, neurologists and neurosurgeons), aside from believing in the efficacy of the technology and its potential for improving diagnoses and treatment, often are paid a fee for its use by the patient. Furthermore, they may want to justify the purchase of the technology to hospital administration through high volume. And they may derive professional prestige from the increasing perceived importance of a technology that they control. In the case of MRI, they may be actual investors in the unit. Thus, the specialist, in many instances, is interested in creating demand for the technology by expanding its applications. MRI was believed to have great potential for expanded use (National Institutes of Health, 1987). Unlike technologies such as lithotripsy that have limited applications under specific circumstances, MRI can be used for a wide range of neurological complaints and other selected conditions (although it is not necessarily the most cost-effective modality available). MRI is attractive to investors no doubt in part because of potential applications, including imaging of the heart and differentiation of benign from malignant tissue.

In short, despite the resource constraints faced by hospitals and despite the relatively limited proven clinical applications of MRI when it first arrived on the market, several aspects of the resource environment were favorable to its diffusion, including the level of hospital profits during 1983 to 1985 under PPS; the overall expansionary economic environment, which provided investment opportunities for corporations and for physicians who otherwise may have been feeling an economic pinch; and the potential for generating demand for the technology by expanding its applications. The only serious resource restriction early adopters faced was the initial delay by private insurers and Medicare in determining reimbursement levels for scans. Even this restriction was lifted quickly when Medicare approved payment for MRI scans of the central nervous system in 1986.

Environmental uncertainty has two facets: the difficulty of making accurate predictions about key factors of concern to an organization, such as the demand for a new product or the impact of changes in a government policy; and the lack of control an organization has over key aspects of the environment (for example, interest rates) even if it can predict what will happen with some accuracy. Uncertainty is characterized by both breadth (the number of variables that are unpredictable or uncontrollable) and intensity (the degree of uncertainty and the importance of the variables) (Thompson, 1967). An organization facing uncertainty may pursue a variety of risk-reduction strategies, including trying to increase control of the environment (vertical integration), to reduce individual risk (joint ventures or consortia), and to make the environment predictable (the great consultant explosion).

In the 1980s the uncertainty hospitals experienced with the imposition of PPS and other government policies, such as delays in determining a capital pass-through policy (how capital needs would be treated by federal payers) and changes in tax laws and CON regulations, was exacerbated by the unprecedented restructuring in the hospital sector these changes triggered. In addition, many hospitals perceived PPS as the first step in establishing a capitated (that is, prospective reimbursement per person per time period) payment system in the entire health sector, especially as HMOs, with the encouragement of the federal government, continued to increase their market shares aggressively in many areas. One of the effects of this uncertainty was to change the long-standing relationship between hospital administration, which now was deeply concerned about cutting costs, and hospital medical staff, which generally was accustomed to a great deal of autonomy in making treatment decisions. Strains appeared around a number of issues, including technology acquisition, the use of hospital resources, and the best way to treat patients. In effect, hospitals and other health providers were facing an environment in the throes of a transformation that significantly altered long-standing relationships and expectations (Glandon and Morrisey, 1986; Custer, Moser, Musacchio, and Wilkens, 1988).

With regard to MRI specifically, some industry insiders speculated that the federal government intentionally exacerbated uncertainty with its lengthy delays in making key decisions on reimbursement levels for MRI outpatient scans and capital pass-through policy for hospitals. Other aspects of uncertainty, which had nothing to do with government policy, were concerns about the efficacy of the technology for applications beyond those concerned with the central nervous system and concerns about the survivability of manufacturers and about early obsolescence (Hillman and Schwartz, 1986; Kimberly and others, 1989). Here the experience with computed-tomography (CT) scanners is instructive. Early adopters of CTs experienced two problems. First, the early generation of machines quickly became obsolete because of rapid advances in the technology. Second, General Electric, which entered the CT market relatively late, soon captured the lion's share of the market with its newer, more sophisticated equipment. Early adopters found that they had to buy entirely new machines because General Electric either could not or would not upgrade earlier machines. Although MRI was designed to allow for upgrading, a well-founded concern about early obsolescence remained. Furthermore, by early 1986 there were six major manufacturers (later reduced to five) and several smaller manufacturing companies in the MRI market. These manufacturers were producing units with permanent, resistive, and superconducting magnets of strengths ranging from 0.15 to 2.0 tesla (Teplensky, Kimberly, Hillman, and Schwartz, 1989). Decision makers needed to determine not only whether MRI was clinically efficacious but also which manufacturer and which configuration (tesla, magnetic type, and software) would best meet their needs and would survive in a competitive market place.

In the immediate term, most of these uncertainty factors affected hospitals more profoundly than individual physicians for several reasons. First, many of the government cost-containment policies were directed specifically at hospitals. Second, hospitals, being bureaucratic organizations, faced numerous internal obstacles to responding quickly to opportunities and constraints; these obstacles included their standard operating procedures and their strong preference for controlling technology whenever possible. Third, hospitals, more than individual physicians, remembered the CT experience because they had had to pay the price of early obsolescence. Fourth, hospital administrators, again much more than physicians, had doubts about the efficacy of the technology (Kimberly and others, 1989). Under such circumstances the traditional method of acquisition, outright purchase, appeared highly risky to many hospitals, except those teaching hospitals that considered it part of their mission to have the latest technology (and that were often provided with research subsidies by manufacturers). Two risk-reduction strategies were available in the early years of diffusion: a wait-and-see approach or formation of some kind of joint venture or consortium.

The proclivity for the wait-and-see approach (in some instances imposed by state CON requirements) created the opportunity for physician ventures, which claimed a large share of the MRI market by the end of 1986. Radiologists and neurologists had the expertise to operate and the conviction to commit themselves to the technology early on. Not being constrained by the need to get approval from a board, they could act as soon as a group of investors was identified. Most physician-investors first attempted to get access to an MRI unit through their hospitals but at signs of hesitation or delay concomitantly began exploring other avenues of acquisition (Kimberly and others, 1989). Because many physician ventures were made up of neurologists and radiologists, they had an established referral base that was likely to remain stable even if hospitals subsequently opened units. Even so, physician-investors were interested in minimizing their risks. Most groups consisted of multiple investors who put up reasonably small amounts of money, tended to opt for lease/purchase agreements, and often arranged to put their units on hospital grounds.

In summary, all health care providers work within the same general environment, one that was characterized in the 1980s by rapid and, in many respects, unpredictable change. Specific components of that environment, however, affect different providers in different ways, posing overwhelming obstacles for some, minor constraints for others, and opportunities for still others. One might predict that in a highly uncertain environment providers would defer risky decisions. Such seems to have been the case, at least initially, for the vast majority of hospitals, including almost half the members of the Council of Teaching Hospitals. Deferral by hospitals created an opportunity for physician-investors. Nonetheless, by the end of 1987 hospitals had once again become, proportionately, the dominant investors in MRI technology. Two factors contributed to this evolution: the competitive situation, which both increased uncertainty and increased pressures to act to ensure organizational survival, and the development of new, low-risk acquisition alternatives.

Competition, a central variable in ecological analysis, may help explain not only why a technology might or might not be adopted but also the pattern of diffusion in local markets. Organizational ecologists typically define competition relatively narrowly with survival being the dependent variable (Hannan and Freeman, 1984). In this definition the intensity of competition is a function of the number of competitors and the level of demand. The competitive dynamics of a market depend on competitors' key characteristics (size, generalist-versus-specialist orientation, price competition-versus-diversification strategies), the degree of uncertainty they face, and the resources they have available. These factors then affect configurations of organizations at the community level in consistent ways (the principle of isomorphism). The analysis of competitive dynamics in local markets presents a substantial challenge for researchers and, to date, has been neglected in the empirical literature on organizational ecology. The analysis of MRI diffusion presents an opportunity to explore these dynamics empirically.

Research in organizational ecology up to this point has concentrated on analyzing competition among the same types of organizations (restaurants, newspapers), although some studies have treated variations as different "species" (seasonal versus year-round restaurants, dailies versus special-interest weeklies). In the case of MRI, several different types of organizations are adopting the technology—hospitals, physician groups, hospital/physician joint ventures, and intermediary organizations. Not only is each type of organization competing with like organizations, but the different types of organizations are competing with each other. In addition, other competitive relationships among health care providers affect the rate and pattern of MRI diffusion. In short, the competitive environment is quite complex, although it may be no more or less complex than other environments were they carefully analyzed.

Much competition occurs among hospitals for patients and physicians within a given market area. The nature and intensity of that competition depend on such factors as the size of the hospitals; their financial situations; their areas of expertise; and the size, demographics, and geographical concentration of their patient base and physician population. For example, we would expect that a market area that has a mix of small, medium, and large hospitals (as defined by number of beds) will have a different competitive dynamic from one in which all the hospitals are roughly the same size. In the mixed market there may be intense competition between hospitals of roughly the same size, while in the homogenous market there may be intense competition among all the hospitals. Likewise, two market areas that have a similar composition of hospital population probably will have different competitive dynamics if one is characterized by a declining population and low per capita income and the other by a growing population and an expanding economy.

Competition also exists between hospitals and health maintenance and preferred-provider organizations and outpatient facilities. Here, the timing and rate of penetration by these new providers and facilities are important. Take, for example, two communities (A and B) that are similar in number and mix of hospitals and key demographic variables. Community A has six, well-established HMOs that have been operating for several years and consistently account for approximately 35 percent of the insurance market. In Community B six HMOs have entered the market within the last two years; they have quickly claimed 35 percent of the insurance market and are aggressively trying to expand their market shares. The providers in Community B are confronted not only by increased competition but also by increased uncertainty because they do not have much experience in dealing with HMOs, it is not clear how much of the market HMOs will ultimately claim, and it is clear that all the HMOs will survive.

Competition among physicians is also a factor—specifically, in the case of MRI, competition between radiologists and hospital radiology groups. Hospitals located in markets in which there is a glut of radiologists may be in a better position to defer technology-acquisition decisions than those that have few radiologists. At the same time, it is in just such markets that radiologists may be looking for investment opportunities and ways to set themselves apart from other radiologists.

The ways that variations in competitive intensity affect either the rate or pattern of diffusion are, at present, unclear. Precise impacts remain to be determined through further analysis. MRI units, however, tend to enter the market in clusters. In almost every Standard Metropolitan Statistical Area for which we have data, several units opened within twelve months after the first unit was established. This diffusion pattern raises the question of whether the ownership arrangement of the first unit influences subsequent diffusion and what factors account for the timing of the first unit.

Beyond the competitive relationships in the local market area, two sets of competitive relationships at the national or regional level are important. One is the nature of competition among MRI manufacturers and the other is competition among MRI intermediaries. By early 1986 there were six major MRI manufacturers. As they competed for market share, considerable opportunities for potential purchasers were created. By mid-1987 one manufacturer had been acquired by another large manufacturer, allowing the acquirer to achieve dominance in the market. In addition, several mergers by other manufacturers had occurred, and about half a dozen small manufacturers had entered the market. Manufacturers' strategies, particularly regarding which states and what sort of clientele to target and which products to offer, have had a discernible impact on both the rate and pattern of diffusion (Teplensky, Kimberly, Hillman, and Schwartz, 1989).

Likewise, the number, types, and strategies of intermediaries have also affected the pattern of MRI acquisition. On the one hand, intermediaries acted to facilitate acquisition by either hospital or nonhospital investors by providing financing, managerial expertise, or physical plant (singly or in combination). On the other hand, rumor of their entry into a market was an additional competitive threat to hospitals, which frequently responded by quickly acquiring their own units as a defensive maneuver. Hospitals that originally rejected the idea of a joint venture with physicians reconsidered once the physicians contacted an intermediary group (Kimberly and others, 1989).

The environmental factors noted all have influenced the diffusion of MRI. We do not know yet the relative importance of each, how they interact, and if they affect behavior in consistent ways. Because the situation is complicated by a multiplicity of actors and the number of questions we are interested in answering, it is useful to divide the overall problem into manageable parts. A means of doing so would be to pose three broad questions: Under what circumstances do hospitals buy a unit or enter a consortium or joint venture or lease a unit? Under what circumstances do freestanding sites enter a market? Do similar patterns of ownership characterize similar market areas over the long term? The first question is in the purview of traditional diffusion theory. The second question is most productively approached through ecological analysis. The last question deals with community demographics but also is an extension of ecological analysis insofar as we are looking at organizational variation rather than organizational transformation or failure.

Limitations of Organization Ecology in Explaining MRI Diffusion

Organizational ecology is not without its own limitations. Campbell (1969) proposes that the process of organizational change is essentially imitative. It moves from organizational variation to selection by the environment to retention by the organization and finally to diffusion to other organizations. In this process, the environment determines which organizational forms survive. However, reviewing the evidence from MRI nationwide, we find similar diffusion patterns in dissimilar market areas and dissimilar diffusion patterns in similar market areas. Should we find, when our analyses are completed, that local environmental variations do not have as much of an impact as ecological theory might predict, there may be two explanations.

First, the combination of unusually intense competition in an unusually uncertain environment may explain a more limited impact of environmental factors than predicted. Because of competitive pressures, some decision makers feel there is no time to observe the success or lack of success of a competitor's latest initiative. Rather, variation is followed by diffusion, without the intermediate evaluative steps; organizations do not wait to see whether the environment selects a variation, they simply act. Second, national contacts may override local conditions. For example, a hospital chain may have a national policy regarding technology acquisition that restricts local choices regardless of conditions in the community. Another aspect is the dramatic growth of the health care industry and hospitals' reliance on it. Many consultants, despite careful consideration of local conditions, have preferred solutions and may push hospitals in these directions. A more important example in the case of MRI is the national communications network of neurologists and radiologists. A radiologist from California can tell radiologists from places as diverse as Alabama, Minnesota, and Texas about the performance of her MRI venture. They, in turn, may start similar ventures, despite tremendous differences in market area.

As Betton and Dess (1985, p. 756) observe, population ecologists have become so preoccupied with the process of selection, they have neglected the far more common process of variation, thereby artificially limiting the application of organization ecology. By focusing on entry and exit, theorists neglect the process of adaptation through variation, a central concern of population ecology in the biological sciences. In short, important factors apart from local environmental conditions may account for entry of freestanding imaging organizations into markets or adoption decisions by hospitals. Unfortunately some of the factors, such as physician contacts with other physicians or the specifics of hospital/consultant relationships, are not easily measured. One might still argue that, over the long term, ventures that do not reflect the realities of the environment will fail, but this is not necessarily the case either. First, hospitals are quite capable of operating at least some of their services at a loss for extended periods of time. Second, if the applications of MRI in fact expand significantly, units that were bad investments at one time may be perfectly viable at a later time.

Thus, we may not be able to delineate the relationships among uncertainty, munificence, competition, and specific configurations of units. In the short run, other factors, such as organizational or individual learning, may override expected outcomes. In the long run, the diffusion process and the health care environment are both evolving so rapidly that it will be difficult to determine what organizational form was the best "fit" at any one time. In many respects, this and the other problems mentioned in this section are not unlike those confronting researchers engaged in the empirical analysis of any complex social phenomenon, regardless of the paradigm they choose as their framework.

The difficulties in choosing the appropriate organizational form(s) for providing MRI services can be ameliorated if we do not restrict ourselves to the criterion of survival. Rather, in evaluating "goodness of fit" with the environment, we might want to establish other criteria, such as profitability or the ability to delivery quality care efficiently. The ability to deliver quality care, especially, would introduce a normative element to population ecology that has been missing; the lack of such a normative element makes much of the existing empirical work, in our view, less interesting than it might be.

Our next challenge is to determine the ways in which environmental variations within market areas influence rates and patterns of diffusion and the long-term survival of units, keeping in mind the multidimensional nature of the environment and the interplay of national influences and local conditions. The results of these analyses will help us determine just how useful our efforts to infuse diffusion theory with ecological analysis are.

References

Aldrich, H., and Stern, R. "Resource Mobilization and the Creation of U.S. Producers' Cooperatives 1835-1935." *Economic and Industrial Democracy*, 1983, *4*, 371-406.

Alexander, J. A., Kaluzny, A. D., and Middleton, S. C. "Organizational Growth, Survival and Death in the U.S. Hospital Industry: A Population Ecology Perspective." *Social Science and Medicine*, 1986, *22* (1), 303–308.

Andersen, J. G., and Jay, S. J. "Computers and Clinical Judgements: The Role of Physician Networks." *Social Science and Medicine*, 1985, *20* (10), 969–979.

Anderson, G. F., and Steinberg, E. "To Buy or Not to Buy: Technology Acquisition Under Prospective Payment." *New England Journal of Medicine*, 1984, *311*, 182–185.

Astley, W. G., and Fombrun, C. J. "Collective Strategy: Social Ecology of Organizational Environments." *Academy of Management Review*, 1984, *8*, 576–587.

Becker, D. M., Sarel, D., and Gardner, L. B. "Decision to Adopt New Medical Technology: A Case Study of Thrombolytic Therapy." *Social Science and Medicine*, 1985, *21* (3), 291–298.

Becker, M. H. "Factors Affecting the Diffusion of Innovation Among Health Professionals." *American Journal of Public Health*, 1970, *60*, 294–304.

Betton, J., and Dess, G. "The Application of Population Ecology Models to the Study of Organizations." *Academy of Management Review*, 1985, *10* (4), 750–757.

Brittain, J. W., and Freeman, J. "Organizational Proliferation and Density-Dependent Selection." In J. Kimberly and R. Miles (eds.), *Organizational Life Cycles*. San Francisco: Jossey-Bass, 1980.

Brittain, J. W., and Wholey, D. R. "Organizational Ecology: Findings and Implications." *Academy of Management Review*, 1986, *11* (3), 513–533.

Campbell, D. "Variation and Selective Retention in Sociocultural Evolution." *General Systems*, 1969, *16*, 69–85.

Carroll, G. R. "Organizational Ecology." *Annual Review of Sociology*, 1984, *10*, 71–93.

Coleman, J. S., Katz, E., and Menzel, H. *Medical Innovation: A Diffusion Study*. Indianapolis, Ind.: Bobbs-Merrill, 1966.

Cromwell, J., Ginsburg, P., Hamilton, D., and Sumner, M. *Incentives and Decisions Underlying Hospitals' Adoption and Utili-*

zation of Major Capital Equipment. Cambridge, Mass.: ABT Associates, 1975.

Cromwell, J. and Kanak, J. R. "The Effects of Prospective Reimbursement Programs on Hospitals and Service Sharing." *Health Care Financing Review,* 1982, *4,* 67–88.

Custer, W. S., Moser, J. W., Musacchio, R. A., and Wilkens, R. D. "Prospective Payment and Hospital-Medical Staff Relationships." In M. V. Pauly and W. K. Kissick (eds.), *Lessons from the First Twenty Years of Medicare.* Philadelphia: University of Pennsylvania Press, 1988.

Davis, K., Andersen, G., and Steinberg, E. "Diagnosis Related Group Prospective Payment: Implications for Health Care and Medical Technology." *Health Policy.* 1984, *4* (2), 139–147.

Delacroix, J., and Carroll, G. R. "Organizational Foundings: An Ecological Study of Newspaper Industries of Argentina and Ireland." *Administrative Sciences Quarterly,* 1983, *28,* 274–291.

Evens, R. G., and Evens, R. G., Jr. "Economic Analysis of MR Imaging Units in the United States in 1987." *Radiology,* 1988, *166,* 27–30.

Evens, R. G., Jost, R. G., and Evens, R. G., Jr. "Economic and Utilization Analysis of Magnetic Resonance Imaging Units in the United States in 1985." *American Journal of Radiology,* 1985, *145,* 393–398.

Feder, J., Hadley, J., and Zuckerman, S. "How Did Medicare's Prospective Payment System Affect Hospitals?" *New England Journal of Medicine,* 1987, *317* (14), 867–873.

Frost, C.E.B. "Physicians and Medical Innovation." *Social Science and Medicine,* 1985, *21* (10), 1193–1198.

Glandon, G. L., and Morrisey, M. A. "Redefining the Hospital-Physician Relationship Under Prospective Payment." *Inquiry,* 1986, *23,* 166–175.

Greer, A. L. "Advances in the Study of Diffusion of Innovations in Health Care Organizations." *Milbank Memorial Fund Quarterly,* 1977, *55,* 505–532.

Greer, A. L. "Medical Technology and Professional Dominance Theory." *Social Science and Medicine,* 1984, *18* (10), 809–818.

Greer, A. L. "The Adoption of Medical Technology: The Hospital's

Three Decision Systems." *International Journal of Technology Assessment and Health Care,* 1985, *1*, (3), 669–680.

Greer, A. L., and Zakhar, A. A. "Patient Leverage Theory Proves to Be False." *Hospitals,* 1979, *53*, 98–106.

Hannan, M. T., and Freeman, J. "The Population Ecology of Organizations." *American Journal of Sociology,* 1977, *82*, 929–964.

Hannan, M. T., and Freeman, J. "Structural Inertia and Organizational Change." *American Sociological Review,* 1984, *49*, 149–164.

Hillman, A. L., and Schwartz, J. S. "The Adoption and Diffusion of CT and MRI in the United States: A Comparative Analysis." *Medical Care,* 1985, *23* (11), 1283–1294.

Hillman, A. L., and Schwartz, J. S. "The Diffusion of MRI: Patterns of Siting and Ownership in an Era of Changing Incentives." *American Journal of Roentgenology,* 1986, *143*, 963–969.

Hurley, R. E., and Kaluzny, A. D. "Organizational Ecology and Health Services Research: New Answers for Old and New Questions." *Medical Care Review,* 1987, *44* (2), 235–255.

Kaluzny, A. D., Veney, J. E., and Gentry, J. T. "Innovations of Health Services: A Comparative Study of Hospitals and Health Departments." In A. D. Kaluzny, J. T. Gentry, and J. E. Veney (eds.), *Innovation in Health Care Organizations: An Issue in Organizational Change.* Monograph Series 4. Chapel Hill: Department of Health Administration, School of Public Health, University of North Carolina, 1974.

Kimberly, J. R. "Hospital Adoption of Innovation: The Role of Integration into External Information Environments." *Journal of Health and Social Behavior,* 1978, *19*, 361–373.

Kimberly, J. R., and Evanisko, M. "Organizational Innovation: The Influence of Individual, Organizational, and Contextual Factors on Hospital Adoption of Technological and Administrative Innovations." *Academy of Management Journal,* 1981, *24* (4), 689–713.

Kimberly, J. R., and others. "Medical Technology Meets DRGs: Acquiring Magnetic Resonance Imaging Under Prospective Payment." In H. P. Brehm and R. M. Mullner (eds.), *Health Care, Technology, and the Competitive Environment.* New York: Praeger, 1989.

Kimberly, J. R. and others. "Rethinking Organizational Innovation." In J. L. Farr and M. West (eds.), *Innovation and Creativity at Work*. New York: Wiley, 1990.

Marple, D. "Technological Innovation and Organizational Survival: A Population Ecology Study of Nineteenth Century American Railroads." *Sociology Quarterly*, 1982, *23*, 107–116.

National Institutes of Health. *Magnetic Resonance Imaging*. Consensus Development Conference Statement, Oct. 26, 1987, *6*.

National Research Council and Institute of Medicine. *Medical Technology and the Health Care System: A Study of the Diffusion of Equipment-Embodied Technology*. Washington, D.C.: National Academy of Sciences, 1979.

Pennings, J. M. "Organizational Birth Frequencies: An Empirical Investigation." *Administrative Sciences Quarterly*, 1982, *27*, 120–144.

Rapoport, J. "Diffusion of Technological Innovations Among Non-Profit Firms: A Case Study of Radioisotopes in U.S. Hospitals." *Journal of Economics and Business*, 1978, *30* (2), 108–118.

Rogers, E. M. *Diffusion of Innovations*. (3rd. ed.) New York: Free Press, 1983.

Romeo, A. A., Wagner, J. L., and Lee, R. H. "Prospective Reimbursement and the Diffusion of New Technologies in Hospitals." *Journal of Health Economics*, 1984, *3* (1), 1–24.

Russell, L. B. *Technology in Hospitals: Medical Advances and Their Diffusion*. Washington, D.C.: Brookings Institution, 1979.

Schwartz, J. S., and others. "MRI: The Diffusion of an Expensive Technology Under Prospective Payment." *Clinical Research*, 1988, *36*, 795A.

Simon, H. A. *Administrative Behavior*. (2nd ed.) New York: Macmillan, 1957.

Sloan, F., Valvona, J., and Perrin, J. "Diffusion of Surgical Technology: An Exploratory Study." *Journal of Health Economics*, 1986, *5* (1), 31–62.

Teplensky, J. D., Kimberly, J. R., Hillman, A. L., and Schwartz, J. S. "Scope, Timing and Strategic Adjustment in Emerging Markets: Manufacturer Strategies and the Case of MRI." Unpublished manuscript, Leonard Davis Institute of Health Economics, University of Pennsylvania, Philadelphia, 1989.

Thompson, J. D. *Organizations in Action.* New York: McGraw-Hill, 1967.

Ulrich, D. "The Population Perspective: Review, Critique, and Relevance." *Human Relations,* 1987, *40,* 137–152.

U.S. Congress, Office of Technology Assessment. *Diagnosis Related Groups (DRGs) and the Medicare Program: Implications for Medical Technology.* Washington, D.C.: U.S. Government Printing Office, 1983.

Young, R. C. "Is Population Ecology a Useful Paradigm for the Study of Organizations?" *American Journal of Sociology,* 1988, *94* (1), 1–24.

8

Explaining Vertical Integration in Health Care:

An Analysis and Synthesis of Transaction-Cost Economics and Strategic-Management Theory

Stephen S. Mick

Why do organizations, particularly health care organizations, integrate vertically? To answer this question I focus on two relatively new, or at least newly articulated, theories, or, less grandly, hypotheses, that purport to explain vertical integration and deintegration. One is transaction-cost economics, most recently espoused by Williamson in a series of articles and books (1971, 1975, 1985; Williamson and Ouchi, 1981). The other is an approach that does not have a formal name but that I shall call the strategic-management theory of vertical integration. It has been discussed most clearly by Harrigan in a no-less convincing series of articles and books (1983, 1984, 1985a, 1985b). The work of Porter also contributes to this theoretical approach (1980, 1985).

More than two theories of vertical integration exist. Williamson himself lists several: theories of domination, market power, technological imperatives, industry life cycle, tax avoidance, and strategic behavior (1985: 123–128). Harrigan's perspective borrows from several of these theories. Transaction-cost economics also parallels, and may even be a subtheory of, the resource-dependence perspective in organization theory. Pfeffer and Salancik (1978, p. 115) state that one way an organization seeks to rationalize relationships with its environment is by growth through merger, one form of which is vertical integration, "a mechanism . . . to restructure their [the organizations'] environmental interdependence in order to stabilize critical exchanges." The incentive for organizations to undertake vertical integration (and other activity) is to reduce uncertainty in order to plan and survive, and to decrease the need to make risky adaptations (Pfeffer and Salancik, 1978, pp. 138–139). Transaction-cost economics is narrower than this view in that it proposes an overriding efficiency logic of vertical integration; this issue is at the heart of this chapter. I compare transaction costs to Harrigan's view because Harrigan offers a completely contradictory paradigm. This is not the case with a comparison of transaction costs and resource dependence, although such a study would be of interest.

Because the two theories—transaction costs and strategic management—make predictions that stand in stark and conflicting contrast to each other, a problem arises not only for organizational analysts interested in theory but also for makers of health policy and for managers. What is one to make of two cogently argued theories that have diametrically opposed prescriptive implications?

To answer this question requires a description of the two approaches and their different explanations of vertical integration. This description will permit speculation on *why* the theories differ. Reference to health care is minimal in the first half of this chapter because I regard it as critical that readers appreciate how divergent these two approaches are. In the second half of the chapter, I propose that the study of health care organizations offers a means of reconciling the approaches. Hence, I beg the reader's indulgence as I untangle these competing and contradictory theoretical statements before launching into the relevance of the health care sector to this dispute.

Vertical Integration Defined

A standard economic definition is that vertical integration "is the organization of production under which a single business unit carries on successive stages in the processing or distribution of a product which is sold by other firms without further processing"

(Blois, 1972, p. 253). Vertical deintegration is the opposite situation, in which one or more successive steps in the production and distribution process do not take place within a single business unit. Organization theorists will find the vertical-integration definition similar to Thompson's (1967, p. 40) formulation: "It [vertical integration] refers to the combination in one organization of successive stages of production; each stage of production uses as its inputs the product of the preceding stage and produces inputs for the following stage."

Williamson's view is nearly the same except that he distinguishes between "mundane" and "exotic" vertical integration— mundane referring to incorporation of successive stages within a core technology, exotic referring to integration into "peripheral or off-site activities—backward integration into basic materials, lateral integration into components, forward integration into distribution, and the like" (Williamson, 1985, p. 105). As a proponent of the strategic-management school, Harrigan defines vertical integration as a situation in which a firm supplies and distributes its own raw materials and output, respectively (Harrigan, 1983, p. 1). These notions suggest a freight-train metaphor, in which one stage of production is linked to the next and so forth. A river is another common metaphor: "Upstream" refers to production units (suppliers) that provide inputs for the focal unit, "downstream" refers to users or distributors of the focal unit's outputs. Hence, at this general level of definition, there is agreement.

Transaction-Cost Economics

The current status of transaction-cost economics can be gleaned, most obviously, by reading Williamson or some of his interpreters (Moe, 1984; Ouchi, 1977). Critical evaluations are found in Francis, Turk, and William (1983), Granovetter (1985), Perrow (1986), and Robins (1987). Transaction costs are the costs of planning, implementing, monitoring, and enforcing exchanges between parties. They are conceptually distinct from production costs, the direct costs of making a good or providing a service (that is, costs of raw materials, machinery, wage labor). Transaction costs can be considered as overhead costs, administrative costs, or indirect costs related to production of a good or provision of a service inside an organization or to the purchase of a good or service made or provided by an outside organization.

Figure 8.1 is a distillation in a causal-modeling framework of the transaction-cost explanation for vertical integration. The basic logic is simple. An interactive group of factors or attributes exogenous to the organization plays on its decision to integrate vertically. These factors are characteristics of the economic markets within which organizations find themselves.

The first of these factors is uncertainty and complexity. Williamson uses these terms in a broad and undifferentiated manner; in fact, they are never clearly defined, a point of great importance to which I shall return. However, the notion is that when the market becomes uncertain and complex, the organization is forced to integrate vertically to enjoy the putative lower costs of intraorganizational decision making. These benefits include the ability to make decisions sequentially, the ability to control processes, and the ability to have convergent goals. All these activities presumably lead to savings on transaction costs. Williamson argues that this set of factors is closely intertwined with the second factor, bounded rationality: When uncertainty and complexity are high, bounded rationality increases.

Bounded rationality refers to the limits on managers' knowledge, a notion Williamson borrows from Simon (1957) and the "satisficing" school. In effect, decision trees that might illuminate rational paths for action cannot be generated. When a certain threshold or boundary of management's rationality is surpassed, vertical integration is the indicated and preferred organizational strategy because vertical organization presumably allows for increased control and a discrete basis for rational action. In a precise sense, bounded rationality is an aspect of managerial decision making. It is not really an attribute of markets. I note this discrepancy now because it will narrow the focus later on the exogenous factors common to both theoretical positions.

Small-numbers bargaining is the third aspect of the organization's environment that produces vertical integration. The benefit for an organization of dealing in markets with large numbers of buyers, suppliers, or distributors is that these entities are forced to

**Figure 8.1. Transaction-Cost Theory: Causes and Outcomes
of Vertical Integration.**

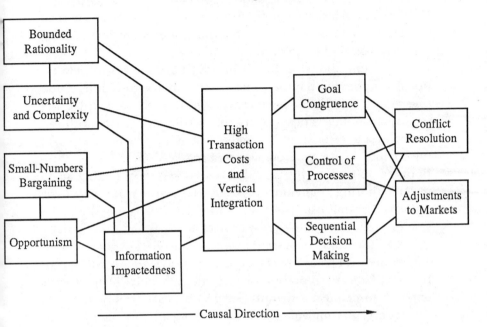

——————— Causal Direction ——————➤

offer competitive prices or high quality or both. When the market
for a good or service is dominated by a small number of buyers,
suppliers, or distributors, the organization may fail to obtain comparable prices and quality for an important reason.

That reason is the fourth factor: opportunism, or misrepresentation by the partner in the market-exchange relationship. Such
misrepresentation need not be malicious, but it can be. Opportunism is most likely to occur under conditions of small-numbers
bargaining, where the focal organization no longer has the ability
to make its exchanges in ideal competitive markets. Opportunism
appears to be omnipresent, but it tends to be more of a force in
small-numbers markets than in competitive ones.

These four factors, but particularly opportunism and environmental uncertainty and complexity, combine to produce *information
impactedness,* a term Williamson uses to describe a state "in which
one of the parties to an exchange is much better informed than is the

other regarding underlying conditions germane to the trade, and the second party cannot achieve information parity except at great cost" (1975, p. 14). When these imbalances in the availability of information are extreme, costs of transactions can be lessened by internalizing the exchanges through vertical integration.

In sum, limits on the ability of administrators to plan rationally (information impactedness) will lead to vertical integration (Fig. 8.1). These limits are affected by insufficient knowledge and inadequate numbers of suppliers and distributors, by opportunism and malfeasance of suppliers and distributors, by complexity and uncertainty in the environment and markets. Overcoming these limits exacts such high transaction costs (the costs of seeking, making, monitoring, and enforcing contracts) that it is less expensive to incur the administrative costs of internally managing the provision or production of the given services or goods.

Williamson contends that the advantages are goal congruence, sequential planning and decision making, and increased control. Williamson proposes that inside vertically integrated as opposed to deintegrated units, subgroup goals are less likely to subvert organizationwide goals, internal organization as a planned system can be more effectively audited than markets, and internal organizational disputes are more easily settled (Williamson, 1975, p. 29). He downplays the barriers to, and subsequent transaction costs of, internal organizational exchanges. By understating the costs of overcoming information impactedness inside organizational structures, Williamson may overstate the benefits of vertical integration, a point made with great vigor by Perrow (1981).

Williamson pays little attention to deintegration, but the model in Figure 8.1 contains an implicit hypothesis: Assuming that the factors on the left-hand side lessen in salience or that the costs of administering the vertically integrated organization become too high, there will be an incentive to deintegrate vertically.

Strategic-Management Theory

Let us begin with Porter. He writes that "[a] challenger may employ integration or deintegration as a means of attacking a leader" (1985, p. 524). This language is completely different from anything found in transaction-cost economics and gives a hint at the conceptual gulf between the two approaches. Porter argues that through vertical integration a nondominant firm can gain advantage in a market even though the transaction (and production) costs within the vertically integrated structure may be higher than those in the market, although they need not be. Harrigan is explicit on this point: "In some cases, effective vertical integration may even require temporary subsidization of one business unit at the expense of the other" (1984, p. 638).

Why a firm (or a hospital) might be willing to subsidize money-losing units (that is, to incur higher production and transaction costs) relates to Harrigan's overall view of vertical integration as management's attempt to control or avoid risks to the central business of the organization by undercutting competition, becoming a technological leader, securing stable inputs (raw materials, capital, labor, patients), developing creative synergies among integrated units, and so forth. Thus, Harrigan's theory stresses management's strategic use of vertical integration in almost complete contradiction to the efficiency-maximization thesis of transaction-cost economics.

This difference becomes clear when we examine the specific points of Harrigan's model and its five variables: demand uncertainty, volatility of competition, bargaining power, corporate-strategy needs, and industry evolution (Figure 8.2). (Unlike the Williamson model, the Harrigan model does not show the consequences of vertical integration. They are so legion and complex that a simple model could not depict them. Because my focus is on the determinants of vertical integration, I feel justified in omitting them.)

Harrigan's first variable is demand uncertainty. When demand is stable, we can expect integration because an organization's sales can increase to absorb the output of adjacent plants without producing "costly excess-capacity penalties." In Harrigan's words, "[B]ecause it would take time for . . . sales growth to occur, one would not expect firms within many embryonic industries (as well as declining industries) to be broadly integrated or engaged in many stages of integrated operations" (1984, p. 644). If demand for a new or declining firm's products is highly uncertain, management can-

Figure 8.2. Strategic-Management Theory: Causes of Vertical Integration.

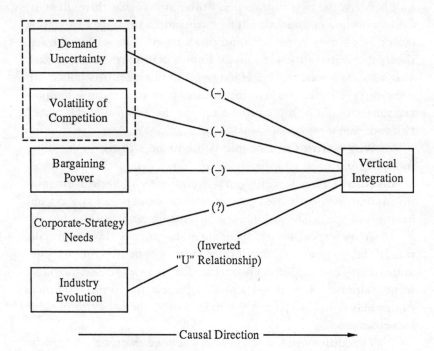

not be certain whether there will be consumer acceptance of new products or new generations of products. Hence, the risks of extending the organization into vertical arrangements do not outweigh the possible benefits. This conclusion is in contradistinction to that of transaction-cost economics, which argues that uncertainty in markets should favor vertical integration because of the resultant lower transaction costs. Neither model considers the possibility that organizations may, in fact, contribute to their environmental uncertainty as a strategic option intended to enhance performance (Jauch and Kraft, 1986), but this is a subject for another article.

The second factor is volatility of competition. Harrigan's proposition is that "the greatest number of successful linked stages and the greatest successful breadths of integrated activities would be expected in settings in which competition is stable" (1984, p. 647). Her notion is that where price warfare and depressed profit margins exist, competition is likely to employ tactics that "devastate" long-term profitability and "sap" innovation. Harrigan lists the elements of industry structure that are important in assessing the volatility of a market: product traits, supplier traits, consumer traits, manufacturing-technology traits, and competitor traits. They form a matrix that tends to be inimical to vertical integration—a chain of linked activities—because, like a wagon train crossing the prairie, an extremely vertically integrated organization is vulnerable to attack, communicates poorly from one end to the next, and responds slowly to the next challenge. By contrast, in turbulent settings, a deintegrated organization can be defended from attack, can communicate accurately, and can change tactics quickly.

Harrigan's writing is not consistent in differentiating between demand uncertainty and volatility, and in one publication (1983) she refers only to volatility. In this chapter, I tend to refer to both these factors as a single one, using Williamson's rubric of uncertainty. This usage will facilitate comparisons between the two theories.

The third factor is bargaining power. When an organization has a great degree of power in a market, it can persuade other organizations to supply inputs or distribute outputs if these are tasks it wishes to avoid doing itself. The characteristics of an organization with high bargaining power are, first, having a product that is specific to an industry and for which no substitutes are available; second, having alternative outlets or sources of supplies; third, already having the ability to make the good or provide the service in question; and, fourth, having dependent suppliers and distributors. Harrigan warns that if an organization does not possess the requisite bargaining power vis-à-vis its suppliers and distributors, and if competition is volatile, vertical integration could be disastrous.

The next, and fourth, factor is corporate-strategy needs. In this instance, the preceding propositions can be nullified by the organization's long-term strategic plans. Harrigan writes: "Vertical integration may be part of a larger strategy involving shared resources and experience curve economies for some businesses, for example, requiring the firm to sustain relationships that [the] strategy framework otherwise would not recommend" (1984, p. 649). These long-term strategies include improving synergies for the entire firm, although one or two subunits might be penalized in the process; and creating technological leadership. The gist is that if particular strategic plans so dictate, the general perils of vertical integration may be seen as risks that must be taken.

The fifth, and final, factor is industry evolution or phase of industry development. The proposition here is that at the early, or embryonic, phase and the late, so-called end-game, phase of the development of an industry, it is unwise to integrate vertically. By contrast, in the intermediate phases vertical integration may be warranted. Here, Harrigan injects some historical perspective into her model. Her numerous observations of different industries lead her to argue that embryonic industries should not risk their venture capital through exposure to the potential vicissitudes in the environment. However, as the industry emerges into some order, imbalances between supplier and distributor firms tend to decrease, learning in the focal organizations has increased, and demand can be expected to exceed the depreciable life of assets. Then vertical integration may help a firm develop innovative processes, devise technological substitutes for labor, maintain secrecy about nonpatentable production processes, and design specialized products and services tailored to the firm's needs.

At the next phase, in which firms are established, scale economies through vertical integration might be desirable. Additionally, more refined management analysis such as forecasting activity levels and measuring value added are undertaken. However, Harrigan warns against overinvolvement in vertical integration at this stage. An organization should not foreclose the potential for deintegration (Harrigan, 1983, p. 25). All the perils already noted apply in full force as the industry moves to a stage in which most organizations are deintegrating, reducing the scope of operations, and even leaving the business entirely. An organization can be burdened with unwieldy structures, lack of flexibility, excess capacity and inventory, high exit costs, and even regulatory barriers prohibiting exit from the market.

In sum, although Harrigan's theory contains a broader array of forces affecting vertical integration than does Williamson's transaction-cost theory, the major features of each are contradictory, specifically in their assessments of how uncertainty and complexity (roughly corresponding to demand uncertainty and volatility of competition in Harrigan) affect the organization's decision to integrate. Harrigan's addition of several other factors, notably bargaining power and corporate-strategy needs, underscores their different approaches, as the next section makes clear.

Why Do the Two Theories Differ?

Taken alone, each theory features compelling rationales for and against vertical integration. Why do they differ in their conclusions?

Differing Definitions of Vertical Integration. The first possible explanation of the difference is that the two approaches are talking about different phenomena; in short, vertical integration means different things in each theory. (I thank Timothy Armstrong for suggesting this explanation to me.) I suggested previously in this chapter that their definitions are similar, and, in general, the two are talking about the same class of phenomena. However, a close reading of Williamson and of Harrigan shows that each emphasizes different aspects of vertical integration.

Williamson's manifest definition fits the usual view of economists. But Williamson's concern is with the exchange process itself, not with the organizational structure. His interest lies in developing, implementing, monitoring, and enforcing implicit and explicit contracts between and among different people and entities. When conditions in a market render the exchange too costly to accomplish, it is time to meld the contracting organizations so that the exchange occurs under new, less costly circumstances. This melding happens to result in vertical integration.

If the transaction itself is viewed as the critical unit of analysis, then the implication is that there is no particular usefulness to the notions of organizational boundary and organizational environment. Barney and Ouchi go one step further: "There is no such thing as an 'organization's structure,' at least as this concept traditionally has been used. Rather, exchanges are governed in a wide variety of ways, using competition or cooperation, rules or trust, and bureaucracies or clans, all simultaneously" (1986, p. 434). Hence, where an organization theorist sees an organization, the transaction-cost economist sees a nexus of contracts, a bundle of exchanges that take place concurrently inside and outside of a mix of organizational forms or governance structures, quasi markets, and markets.

Hence, a dissection of types of vertical-integration structures, a task that is central to Harrigan's work, is neither attempted nor accorded much significance. The emphasis is on a search for the conditions under which a rational organization substitutes "nonmarket administrative relationships for cross-firm market relationships by annexing other organizations operating at different stages of production or distribution" (Moe, 1984, p. 752).

If Williamson is abstract about vertical integration, Harrigan is concrete. The interested reader will find carefully developed depictions of vertical integration in several publications (Harrigan, 1983, 1984, 1985a, 1985b). Harrigan differentiates among breadth, stage, degree of internal transfers, and form of ownership—a paradigm that both Clement (1988) and Mick and Conrad (1988) use in their discussions of vertical integration in health care organizations. Harrigan's point is that many different forms of vertical integration are possible and that there is a correspondence between certain constellations of vertical integration and organizational performance. A unitary, simple definition is inappropriate and defies reality. Harrigan, in the spirit of organizational contingency theory, writes that "the key to successful use of vertical integration is determining how broadly integrated the firm should be at a particular time, how many stages of production to engage in, how much of each task should be done internally, and what form the venture should take. . . . No particular degree, breadth, stage, or form of vertical integration is best for all firms under all circumstances (1983, p. 2). Hence, Harrigan's research effort has been to determine the kinds of vertical integration (and deintegration) that are appropriate in light of the organization's particular objectives and circumstances.

Differing Views of Organizations. A second way Harrigan and Williamson depart from each other is in their portrayals of organizations. If Williamson tends to downplay organizations as organizations and the importance of their boundaries with environments, Harrigan is clearly in the opposite camp. This point is clear in her criticism of the transaction-cost theorists: "They do not go far enough in developing investment ramifications to be useful to managers because they ignore the realities of industry structure and corporate strategies. In brief, economic treatments of market failure de-emphasize the activities of firms that used means other than vertical integration to overcome the information gap this theory describes. Thus, they ignore different firms' interesting and useful strategic responses to market imperfections" (1983, p. 7).

Embedded in Harrigan's perspective is the belief that organizations and their boundaries are real and that what managers do in them matters. The exchanges in which organizations involve themselves are real too, but they are the consequences of organizational activity, decision making, and strategic planning.

Differing Views of Uncertain and Complex Environments. Another possibility for the two theories' opposing predictions is that they view the environment differently. In particular, they have different ways of defining uncertain and complex environments. Williamson's work, not surprisingly given the discussion about his focus on the transaction itself, is vague in this regard. He devotes less than two pages to a discussion of the two adjectives *uncertain* and *complex* in his *Markets and Hierarchies* (1975) and about three pages in *The Economic Institutions of Capitalism* (1985). He uses the endless moves in chess to express the notion of complexity; for uncertainty, he provides no clear definition and notes that high uncertainty means that complete decision trees for action cannot be generated. However, Williamson does identify a source of uncertainty: the opportunism of individuals engaged in exchanges. He writes, "Even if it were possible to characterize the general propensity of a population to behave opportunistically in advance and perhaps even to screen for trustworthiness, knowing that one is dealing with a trader who comes from one part of the opportunism distribution rather than another does not fully describe the uncertainties that arise on this account" (1985, p. 58).

The reader may remember that opportunism is one of the four factors included in the transaction-cost model depicted in Figure 8.1. But for Williamson opportunism is a major source of uncertainty, not a separate factor influencing the vertical-integration decision. He calls opportunism "behavioral uncertainty" and links it to the surprises people cause and to their endless capacity for tricking partners in transactions. Understanding Williamson's view is essential: There is no actual depiction of the environment as such, no view of the environment apart from opportunism. Even in the case of small-numbers bargaining, in which markets with just a few players are compared with those with many players, the focus is on the greater probability that opportunism will affect the focal organization.

Contrast this view to the numerous efforts of organizational analysts to catalog and categorize environmental complexity and uncertainty as well as to use these schemes in empirical research. (See Evan, 1978, and Karpik, 1978, for useful surveys.) For an organization theorist, the type of environment one is talking about is often crucial. Harrigan follows this tradition. In *Strategies for Vertical Integration* (1983), she is fastidious in describing factors that contribute to an environment's volatility (as contrasted to stability). Her volatile environment includes one in which several firms from different groups serve the same customer group; signaling of competitive intentions has been vague or poor; fringe competitors use price cutting to increase their productive capacity; fringe competitors use price cutting below their costs because they themselves cannot deintegrate or take any other actions to reduce their overhead; high product differentiation, frequent process innovations, low consumer switching costs, or lack of product loyalty exist. She concludes: "Thin profitability and rounds of price-cutting are outward signs that competition is volatile within the industry, and patterns of erratic demand signal that imbalances exist in upstream and downstream units as well as units operating within the troubled industry" (1983, p. 32).

By contrast, a nonvolatile, or stable, environment is one that has, according to Harrigan, low product differentiation, infrequent product improvements, high customer switching costs, few strategic groups, clear competitive signals, little history of price competition, and "where all major firms are similarly integrated and recognize their interdependence with respect to the activities of competitors" (1983, p. 32). She states unequivocally the relationship between volatility and vertical integration: "Less internal integration is appropriate under conditions of high uncertainty, volatility, and frequent product modification. More internal integration is appropriate when industry conditions are less volátile and uncertain" (1983, p. 33).

She provides details on industry after industry to make her point about appropriate and inappropriate fit between integration and deintegration and market conditions. In *Strategic Flexibility* (1985a, pp. 163-169), Harrigan graphically illustrates the environmental circumstances that make certain combinations of the four dimensions of vertical integration—breadth, stage, degree of internal transfers, form of ownership—more or less appropriate for a firm.

There is a stark contrast between the detail provided by Harrigan, only a small fraction of which is presented here, and the vague depiction given by Williamson. Underlying this difference may be an important conceptual variance between the two. Williamson's uncertainty corresponds most closely to "state uncertainty," which occurs "when [managers] perceive the organizational environment, or a particular component of that environment, to be unpredictable" (Milliken, 1987, p. 136). According to Milliken, two other classes of uncertainty exist: first, "effect uncertainty," or the "inability to predict what the nature of the impact of a future state of the environment or environmental change will be on the organization" and, second, "response uncertainty," or "a lack of knowledge of response options and/or an inability to predict the likely consequences of a response choice" (1987, pp. 136-137). Effect uncertainty does not necessarily indicate that there is confusion about the nature of the environment, only that there is confusion about what the possible consequences will be for the firm. Harrigan employs a hybrid of both effect and response uncertainty. Her five groups of factors, just discussed, reveal that the dimensions of the environment are only too well understood; their uncertain effect on the organization and the uncertain responses available are the issue.

In the case of state uncertainty, Milliken (1987) contends that managers probably will not be able to follow normative, rational decision methods and will be forced to gather information (a potentially wasteful exercise) in an attempt to circumscribe the uncertainty (read as high transaction costs). One response is to protect key functions of the organization; here Milliken cites Thompson's (1967) organizational buffering activities and Cyert and March's (1963) creation of slack resources. These actions can lead to "diversification-type responses" to reduce organizational vulnerability (Milliken, 1987, p. 139).

However, Milliken notes that effect uncertainty is likely to lead to strategic planning and the development of contingency plans. Response uncertainty will be associated with "high levels" of boundary spanning and information gathering to determine the actions of other organizations in the same circumstances. One would also predict use of forecasting techniques for modeling (Milliken, 1987, p. 140). In short, the emphasis is on strategy making and cautious movement: "If the stakes are high and an incorrect response is perceived to be costly, high levels of response uncertainty may have the effect of delaying strategy implementation as possible alternatives are generated and carefully evaluated" (Milliken, 1987, p. 149). This cautiousness fits nicely with Harrigan's message to avoid pitfalls and exposure of organizational resources through vertical-integration schemes in uncertain terrain.

In short, I believe that Williamson and Harrigan differ in two ways in their understanding of uncertainty in the environment: For Williamson, whatever promotes opportunism creates uncertainty; for Harrigan, specific attributes of the competitive sphere create uncertainty. And, for Williamson, uncertainty, as it leads to opportunism, is a feature of the environment itself; for Harrigan, uncertainty derives less from conditions of the environment than from management's inability to predict the effects of environmental change on the organization and the outcomes of organizational responses. The message of her book *Strategic Flexibility* (1985a) is that management needs to be open, flexible, and creative to respond to negative signals from the environment, particularly in the case of vertical integration (pp. 4–5). For Williamson, it appears obvious that vertical integration, among other organizational responses, is a good way to reduce confusion; for Harrigan, vertical integration can be a risky, even foolhardy, venture into the unknown.

Efficiency Versus Power. Williamson assumes and, in fact, explicitly argues (1985, pp. 32, 258) that the primary force affecting organizational exchanges is the search for efficiency. Transaction-cost economics relegates little if any importance to power and power differentials either in market or in intraorganizational exchanges. For Williamson power is an ill-defined and amorphous concept with little analytical value. His criticism of the strategic-management school makes this view evident. Describing that position as having "reference to efforts by dominant firms to take up and maintain advance or preemptive positions and/or to respond punitively to rivals" (1985, p. 128), he dismisses it because it fails to characterize markets that are not already controlled by a dominant firm or oligopolistic industries. In other words, if dominance (or exertion of power) is an accurate description of the behavior of firms in markets, it is a consequence, not a cause, of successful market activity. If firms are efficient in markets and gain further efficiency by integrating vertically, they will gain power. Power, then, is a function or outcome of efficiency. (See the Introduction in Francis, Turk, and William, 1983.)

Harrigan does not involve herself in the efficiency-versus-power debate; rather, she simply assumes that a major reason for firms to engage in vertical integration is to position themselves strategically in relation to their competitors. In describing her model, she uses language that evokes power and struggle. The term *strategy* itself denotes the martial properties of planning, spying, attacking, counterattacking, deceiving, outwitting, winning, losing. Harrigan finds it incomprehensible that power and its exercise might not be relevant in understanding vertical integration; in fact, the reader may recall that bargaining power is one of her five factors in vertical integration.

Summary. On several grounds we find major differences in transaction-cost economics and strategic-management theory. Definitionally, Williamson is concerned with the transaction itself as opposed to the organizational details surrounding it. Harrigan, however, provides us with probably the most fine-grained definition of vertical integration in any literature, and it is clearly structural in content. A corollary is that Williamson's concern for organizations is minimal, whereas Harrigan's organizations are real, living entities in which managers make decisions. For Williamson, exchanges and transactions give rise to organization; in fact, Williamson's position is that were it not for "market failure," organizations would not be needed at all. For Harrigan, the organization permits exchanges to occur. Their views of the environment also differ considerably: Williamson is vague, Harrigan is specific. What does it matter for Williamson what the environment is like? The critical thing is the degree to which opportunism can be engaged in. For Harrigan, the environment can be parceled into dimensions related to the competitive scene. These dimensions have a bearing on whether an organization should consider vertical integration, when it should consider vertical integration, and what type it should consider. Finally, efficiency is the primal force for transaction-cost economics; power, if it exists, is an epiphenomenon. Although Harrigan does not state how primal either power or efficiency is in her scheme, she is clear that at times efficiency is sacrificed for power and that power considerations are elementary in informing vertical-integration decisions.

In sum, these two theorists share little in common in the philosophical stances underlying their discussions of vertical integration. Williamson's views are derived from microeconomic theory and lead to a highly formalized, abstract, sometimes mathematized, deductive approach to organizational life. Harrigan's views are derived from an eclectic, empirically based, inductive approach. It is no surprise that they should vary in their conclusions. How, then, can these theories be useful in explaining vertical integration?

Proposed Synthesis

The approach I take to synthesize these theories consists of broadening the conception of the environment to include more than markets, hypothesizing that one facet of the environment may make integration a logical activity while another facet may favor deintegration, choosing elements from each theory for a general model, and dealing with the special problem of observing decision making based on transaction costs.

Broadened Conception of Environment. As noted previously, the concept of the environment used by Williamson and

Harrigan is restricted to the competitive market within which an organization is located. Williamson's attention is centered on the contingencies of exchanges; Harrigan's, on competing firms. Williamson provides no detail on the environment's content, and Harrigan spends little time on forces other than those emerging from the competing firms.

I propose that an inclusive view of the environment is called for. Helpful in delimiting this view is the broad notion of environmental context (Emery and Trist, 1965) in addition to a narrow focus on the market. I propose a heuristical two-dimensional typology of environmental forces and market actors that can influence a health care organization. Among environmental forces, a health care organization like a hospital or a health maintenance organization contends with reimbursement systems, both conventional (cost-based) and innovative (prospective or capitated or both); with the epidemiology of the population in the service area (for example, the incidence and prevalence of disease and trauma); with the demography of the population; with the general economic state of the service area; with employers and the coalitions; with regulators at the federal, state, and local levels; with political groups and consumer groups. In the market, the following elements in the health care environment can be identified: insurers and third-party payers; independent, autonomous, self-regulating professionals; employees and labor unions; not-for-profit and profit public and private competitors; for-profit suppliers (of durable medical equipment, drugs, services); and employers.

The intersection of these two dimensions creates variously relevant microenvironments for health care organizations. For example, the intersection of a state regulatory body like a rate-setting commission and a hospital's main competitors—other hospitals—could create a relatively stable environment with certainty in pricing of services and in capital expansion. But the intersection of some other state regulatory body like a licensing board and allied health professionals could create an uncertain and volatile environment for the same hospital.

As I have noted, an overall hypothesis is that, depending on the uncertainty, among other dimensions, of a particular microenvironment, integration or deintegration will result. For example, if federal, state, and local regulatory agencies become uncertain about their policies related to the use of interhospital competition to stem rising costs, hospitals might deintegrate, fearful of costly antitrust suits or other efforts to stem what might be seen as restraints to trade. A Harrigan approach would be supported in this instance. Or, as the demography of a region becomes predictable—for example, the population is aging in a steady, predictable way, and insurers are making reimbursement decisions favoring nursing-home care—vertical integration in this case of long-term-care facilities, may become common. Here, a Harrigan approach is again supported.

However, if insurers change premium levels, reimbursement rates, and benefit packages seemingly at random, and regulators equivocate on ways to stabilize these fluctuations, health care organizations might elect to integrate the insurance function into their structures and self-insure their enrollees in managed health care plans. This development would support the Williamson approach. Or if political forces or consumer groups cause turmoil by making malpractice claims that turn into expensive legal settlements and jury awards, and physicians produce uncertainty in the supply of particular specialty practices like obstetrics, health care organizations might try to integrate these specialists into their structures and pay all or part of their malpractice premiums. Again, Williamson would be supported.

To overcome the narrowness of Williamson and Harrigan alone, a broad view of environments is needed, and there are many sources that one can consult for one. Starbuck's (1976) review of the research on this topic is overwhelming in the richness he uncovered in ways to describe environments. Dess and Beard (1984) provide us with a helpful empirical distillation of these notions into three categories: munificence, which is somewhat like carrying capacity in population ecology (Hannan and Freeman, 1989); complexity (Williamson does use this term, but he is really interested in uncertainty); and dynamism (stability and instability). Although the task of empirical analysis is made more difficult by using multiple dimensions, it is probably a more faithful depiction of environmental texture. Hence, I argue that one should use at least these three dimensions, in addition to uncertainty, in describing the potential effect of separate microenvironments in inducing integration or deintegration.

Simultaneity of Vertical Integration and Deintegration in Health Care. These considerations about the effects of microenvironments lead to the second part of my approach: One facet of the environment may favor integration, while another facet favors deintegration. Health care organizations, in fact, are engaging in integration and deintegration activities at the same time in the same environment. Neither Williamson nor Harrigan clearly addresses this phenomenon.

Vertical integration in health care in the 1980s has not followed the standard depiction of the process. On the one hand, health care organizations have been deintegating various services. Despite sunk costs, hospitals, for example, are deintegrating or "unbundling" many services that have traditionally been seen as central to the mission and definition of a hospital. These services include surgical suites, laboratories, and x-ray facilities. As Mick and Conrad (1988) assert, almost nothing, including nursing services, cannot be (and was not during the turbulence of the 1980s) deintegrated from the core hospital unit. These instances are examples of older patterns being abandoned, of services formerly provided in-house being bought from markets.

On the other hand, an immense amount of vertical integration has also been taking place. Some examples include the addition of upstream and downstream units that provide preventive and primary care, traditional acute care, and intermediate care through rehabilitation centers and nursing homes. Health insurance has also been an added feature. Although inclusion of such units tends to mimic the situation in traditional prepaid group practices or health maintenance organizations, adoptions of such services in the 1980s were legion. These instances are examples of innovative expansion into services that formerly were bought in markets (or may not have been provided at all) but now are provided in-house.

The pervasiveness of this simultaneity in health care needs to be emphasized. A typical example of concurrent integration and deintegration in health care serves to underscore the complexity of the issue. An eighty-bed hospital in a semirural county contiguous to a large metropolitan area in a mid-Atlantic state, during the five-year period from 1983 to 1988, underwent the following changes. It contracted with a nurse-registry agency (a firm that provides nursing services) for coverage of the night shift (midnight to 8:00 A.M.) and all Sunday shifts in the acute-care unit. It closed its obstetrics service and drastically reduced its inpatient surgical services. It contracted with a large urban hospital for its laundry services, having decided not to replace its own outdated laundry. It found an entrepreneur interested in leasing its kitchen and now has its cafeteria services operated independently with the contractor totally at risk for any losses but able to enjoy any profits. During this same period, the hospital expanded its ambulatory services considerably by opening an off-site clinic in a joint venture with a physician group; same-day surgery takes place in this clinic as well as primary care. The hospital marketed a mobile health-service team to newly built light industries in a nearby industrial park. It converted half its inpatient beds into a nursing home. And it joined a preferred provider network of hospitals and offers discounts to participating firms' employees. Observers of the health care sector are well aware of these kinds of activities, but they may be less familiar to others.

The existence of concurrent deintegration and integration might be understood by dissecting the environment into its component parts. Different components of the environment may contribute differently to transaction costs. Balakrishnan and Wernerfelt's (1986) study failed to support the transaction-cost hypothesis in regard to technological changes in the environment—that is, where technologies were changing rapidly, creating uncertainty about what innovation would follow next, organizations tended not to integrate vertically, contrary to the Williamsonian view but in accord with Harrigan. However, vertical integration into nontechnologically related activities did occur, following Williamson but not Harrigan. In health care, where there are both a whirlwind of technological change and physician dependence on high-technology medicine, it is unclear that the Balakrishnan and Wernerfelt findings would hold up as well. (Even small, voluntary, not-for-profit hospitals try to stay abreast of each new technological development. However, it is interesting that in the case of magnetic resonance imaging, documented in Chapter Seven, a good deal of contractual activity between hospitals and other entities, particularly medical groups and entrepreneurs, has occurred. There appears to be a blend of both vertical integration and market purchase for the same technology.) But the main point is that Balakrishnan and Wernerfelt's work suggests that theory and research should concentrate on linking variety in the environment with variety in decisions to integrate or deintegrate.

   Salient Elements of Each Theory. What we need then, is a model that can accommodate the simultaneity of vertical integration and deintegration. The previous discussion of differences in Williamson's and Harrigan's explanations implied that each approach was deeply rooted in differences in disciplinary and ontological assumptions. These roots make each approach more extreme than it needs to be because of the requirement that each be faithful to its tradition. I argue that transaction-cost economics and strategic-management theory both need to be disentangled from their philosophical roots and stances and recombined into a single model. Only in this way can we find a satisfactory model that encompasses the diversity and simultaneity of integration and deintegration, at least in the health care sector.

   In an eclectic model, there is no doctrinal reason why management's potential consideration of transaction costs cannot be added to other factors informing the vertical-integration decision. Robins (1987), in his perceptive critique of Williamson's approach, is clear about how transaction-cost thinking widens, but does not replace, strategy formulation necessitated by changing environmental circumstances: "Transaction-cost theory can play an important part in strategy formulation by providing an analytical framework for discussion of the relative cost advantages offered by different forms of organization under specified environmental conditions. . . . Organization [vertical integration] is one competitive factor among many, and its relative importance in business strategy will be determined by the relationships between environmental conditions and the existing structure of the firm. Much of the power of transaction-cost analysis stems from the fact that it can help to clarify the specific conditions that lend strategic importance to organizational design" (1987, pp. 80–81).

   In a combined model, one has the happy prospect of an

enriched and subtle combination of forces on which to base a health care organization's integration decisions. Conrad, Mick, Madden, and Hoare (1988) developed seven testable hypotheses that, in effect, borrowed heavily on the transaction-cost approach but also anticipated the incorporation of other financial and economic factors in the vertical-integration decision. For example, they hypothesized that "vertical integration may occur in response to market barriers caused by imperfections in input markets, regulation, or both" (1988, p. 65). The inclusion of regulation implies that there is benefit in considering a broad spectrum of forces bearing on vertical integration.

Figure 8.3 depicts a model that explicitly incorporates factors other than those linked to transaction costs. The matrix of market actors and environmental forces that I suggested as a way to broaden the concept of the environment becomes the starting point in the new model. Its diversity reflects, I believe, the empirical complexity of the health care environment. The degree to which any of the cells is uncertain, complex, low on munificence, stable or unstable, or some combination of all these, will have an effect on each of the following intermediate group of factors. In this chapter I do not develop hypotheses that refine and specify these relationships, although this is a task that should be undertaken. The point to be emphasized is simply that the environment consists of a multitude of forces influencing an organization and, hence, the factors involved in vertical integration. There are five such factors.

First, the most obvious reason that an organization would integrate is if it leads to economies in production costs. It is ironic that this factor is not discussed in and of itself by either Williamson or Harrigan. In one of the few empirical studies of the transaction-cost model, Walker and Weber found that "the effect of transaction costs on make-or-buy decisions was substantially overshadowed by comparative production costs" (1984, p. 387). Although there may be important boundary conditions to the effect of production costs on vertical integration (for example, the requirement that these costs be simple to measure and be known to all concerned), there is a need to have this factor in any complete model of vertical integration. Second, comparative transaction costs are a potential decision point, as suggested in the preceding section. In trans-

Figure 8.3. Synthesized Transaction-Cost and Strategic-Management Theory of Vertical Integration.

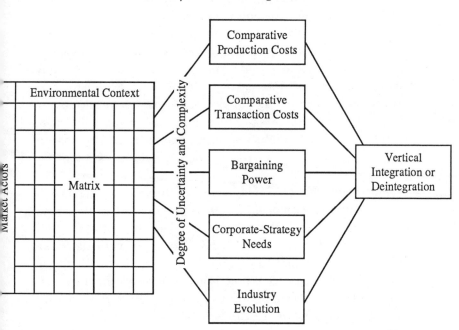

action costs, I include the costs of intraorganizational exchange, which Williamson, as noted, tended to underestimate in his work. Third, Harrigan's bargaining power of the organization is included and is hypothesized to be influenced by the relevant intersection or intersections of market actors and environmental forces. The same is true of Harrigan's corporate-strategy needs, the fourth group in the proposed model. Fifth, the model contains the industry-evolution factor, another from Harrigan's scheme. Where hospitals are in their general evolution may well affect their general propensity to integrate or deintegrate, but the model also points to the possibility that environmental forces could contribute to this evolution.

This model encompasses the variety and simultaneity of vertical integration and deintegration in health care. It implies that the management of a hospital, for example, may consider transaction costs along with its market position in determining whether to integrate vertically. Management may also decide that, despite increased transaction costs and the power it has in the market, it will proceed with vertical integration for long-range strategic reasons. At present, however, health-services researchers and organization theorists are not able to determine the relative weight of any of these factors in decision making. Clearly, however, microenvironments can be arrayed along continua of uncertainty/certainty and complexity/simplicity and their positions on them, in turn, affect the criteria of production costs, transaction costs, market power, corporate-strategy needs, and stage of industry evolution.

Decision Making Based on Transaction Costs. The methodology implied in this model is to test its propositions through first-hand observation or through primary data, or both, on how vertical-integration decisions are made. There are particular problems with the transaction-cost component of this effort. Williamson and Ouchi (1981) and later Williamson (1985), aware that there was a lack of research either supporting or rejecting the transaction-cost paradigm, understood that there was (and is) an unresolved measurement problem. Williamson himself notes that "accounting data, even rather detailed accounting data, are often poorly suited for the needs of transaction cost economics" (1985, p. 104). Research studies employing a transaction-cost approach are not much help either: "Direct measures of transaction costs are rarely attempted" (Williamson, 1985, p. 105). But just because research might determine that transaction-cost logic does not prevail, let alone exist, it does not follow that the theory is wrong. The issue is, If transaction-cost logic were used, would the same integration and deintegration decisions be made?

Williamson confers on organizational analysts a disciplinary advantage of observation that he feels could be a direct test of transaction-cost hypotheses, although, in his view, organizational studies have yet to exploit this advantage (1985, pp. 402–403). This lack of effort is not surprising, however. For a variety of reasons, organizational theorists remain suspicious of transaction-cost economics (Cook, 1977; Francis, Turk, and Williams, 1983; Perrow, 1981, 1986); much of this suspicion stems from the difficulty of measuring transaction costs and of separating transaction costs from production costs. Furthermore, nowhere does Williamson assist researchers by operationally defining transaction costs.

One possible but as yet unused avenue may be found in the research on transfer pricing (Eccles, 1985; Griffith, 1987, pp. 322–323). Transfer prices are those prices charged to one intraorganizational unit for goods or services purchased from another. One typical way these prices are determined is by comparison with the prices of the same goods or services in the market. (Eccles lists three other ways transfer pricing is accomplished; but the important point here is that it is, in fact, possible to account for these prices.) Although the transfer price usually refers to production costs, there is probably an additional or "hidden" administrative or overhead charge that, if carefully accounted for, could be isolated as transaction costs. Hence, an approach is available for researchers that distinguishes between production and transaction costs, and the measurement problem may not be as recalcitrant as some have argued (Perrow, 1986).

Provided that the measurement issue is resolved, organizational analysts could then examine exactly what decision processes lead to vertical integration and to deintegration. Figure 8.4 is a depiction of just the transaction-cost component of the model in Figure 8.3. From the two cost curves shown I derive a number of hypothetical managerial decision-making processes leading to vertical integration. Figure 8.4 concentrates on an increase in environmental uncertainty, the critical area of disagreement between Williamson and Harrigan.

Transaction-cost theory predicts that, for market exchanges, as environmental uncertainty increases, so do transaction costs. I assume that this prediction is also true for internal organizational exchanges but at a decreased rate. Hence, one can draw two transaction-cost curves, one for market-based transactions (m), the other for intraorganizational based (internal) transactions (h), such that

$$d_y/d_{xm} > 0 \quad \text{and} \quad d_y/d_{xh} > 0$$

Under these assumptions, until the intersection of m and h, the transaction costs involved in purchasing a service from the market

Figure 8.4. The Decision to Integrate Vertically.

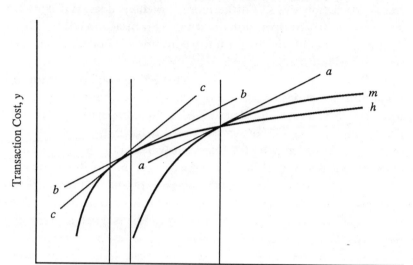

Degree of Environmental Uncertainty, x

are less than those of having the service supplied by the health care organization itself, other things being equal. (In reality, the h curve is hypothetical from the point of view of a manager; it is assumed that the organization is not yet vertically integrated, so there would be no way of knowing what the actual costs of internal transfers would be.) After intersection, the organization would save by producing the service itself.

Figure 8.4 generates several hypotheses. The first is that when transaction costs of market exchanges surpass transaction costs of internal organizational exchanges, an organization will integrate vertically. When the curves m and h intersect, vertical integration will result, which suggests that management will wait until it can achieve a comparative net savings in transaction costs. If comparative cost calculations are made slowly, management may not make a vertical-integration decision until afterward, when m is greater than h.

The second hypothesis is that when transaction costs of market exchanges are less than the costs of internal organizational exchanges but the rate of increase of internal organizational exchange begins to decrease, an organization will integrate vertically. This hypothesis refers to the point at which the slope of h (cc) just begins to decrease (where q_1 *intersects h*). Translated, the transaction costs of internal production of the service are increasing at a diminishing rate, and at some point in the future the marginal cost will be smaller and smaller as the environment becomes increasingly uncertain. A health care manager, surveying the environment and monitoring the costs of market transactions, however roughly, could well note that although market costs are acceptable now and in the near term, the potential transaction costs of internal production might level off enough to make vertical integration a plausible option. The manager, following Mick and Conrad (1988), might have the following thoughts: We've been buying our laundry services from White Sheet, and we should be able to do this for a while longer. But I have the feeling that as the market gets crazier, we'll find that it's going to be harder to do business with White Sheet or anyone else. It's more trouble to do the laundry in-house right now, but this could change. I think we should look seriously at the possibility of doing our own laundry.

The third hypothesis is that when transaction costs of market exchanges are less than the costs of internal organizational exchanges but the rates of increase of both types of cost become equal, an organization will integrate vertically. This hypothesis refers to the situation in which the slope of h (bb) is equal to the slope of m (aa) at the point where m is intersected by h. From there on, the increase in environmental uncertainty leads to a faster decrease in the rate of increase of costs via internal production than via market purchase. Our health care manager might well note that market costs are now closing in on the cost of transacting the exchange internally.

Figure 8.4 implies that these alternative hypotheses are a subset of a larger set of possibilities given different shapes and combinations of market and intraorganizational transaction-cost curves. The three hypotheses just presented are hardly exhaustive. But they do assume that management knows that there are such things as transaction costs and that they are measured, however roughly. The logic of the second and third hypotheses implies more strategic awareness than that of the first hypothesis, but all three assume that management understands that there are costs associated with the alternate activity not presently engaged in—that is, that a nonvertically integrated organization knows something about the transaction costs of vertically integrated organizations. Another issue is that no one knows when management makes the vertical-integration decision as it confronts the converging transaction-cost curves shown in Figure 8.4; for that reason I present three separate hypotheses.

Whatever result hypothesis testing such as this reveals, the researcher would then proceed to the other components of the model in Figure 8.3 and determine the relative influence they do or do not have on the integration outcome. Obviously, these are all sticky empirical questions, but, I submit, they are ones that a thorough test of the transaction-cost model must undertake to answer. Quite clearly, such testing entails a major research effort, which I hope this chapter will help advance.

Implications for Health Care

If researchers were to rely solely on the recommendations of the professional and trade literature on health care management, they would have to reject Williamson's hypotheses and probably accept some version of Harrigan's. (An exception is Jacobson's 1989 case studies of hospital/physician joint ventures, which are explained by transaction-cost economics.) However, there is growing disillusionment with vertical integration in health care, increasing stories of deintegration, and a general reevaluation of where vertical integration has led health care organizations. (See Mick and Conrad, 1988, for a brief review.)

It is a risky, yet enticing, leap to suggest that part of the increasingly high cost of health care is due in part to increases in transaction costs both inside and outside health care organizations. Organizations that are integrated but would have lower transaction costs if they were not, as well as those that are not integrated but would have lower transaction costs if they were, contribute disproportionately to overall system costs. The popularity of strategic management in health care is easy to understand as health care organizations scramble to improve their chances for survival and seek a new rhetoric to demonstrate that they can be run according to the latest business techniques (Stevens, 1989). Hence, it is also easy to see the appeal of a model like Harrigan's, grounded as it is in a broad survey of industries and written in an accessible, prescriptive manner.

Health care managers may too quickly concentrate on Harrigan's corporate-strategy factor in attempting vertical integration and may be willing to wait as long as they can financially until their competitors drop out of the picture or until their own economic situation is in peril. Harrigan's cautious nonintegration-to-deintegration prescription, arising from the environmental factors of demand and uncertainty and competitive volatility, may too easily be ignored. And if integration were accomplished and assets did not become vulnerable as she predicts, this result would seem to confirm Williamson's view that integration in uncertain environments is a way to lower transaction costs.

But the irony is that clear accounting of the transaction costs of vertical integration in uncertain environments might reveal a substratum of wholly unanticipated managerial difficulties. The simple truth is that, apart from experience in prepaid group practices and health maintenance organizations, many health care managers, and their educators, are not trained or experienced in operating vertically integrated systems. And even if they are, no one seems at the present time to have a clear sense of the comparative costs of owning one's own inpatient unit versus contracting with an independent inpatient unit as many health maintenance organizations have. As I noted, one must account for the potentially high internal transaction costs of administering a novel or large (or both) organizational system of vertically integrated parts. Harrigan herself finds fault with Williamson on this point: "Although, as Williamson . . . has suggested, firms may integrate to escape external costs associated with market transactions, there are costs to managing transfers across internal boundaries, as well" (1985a, p. 100).

Thus, although this chapter is an exploration of the conflicts of two theories in explaining vertical integration, it is also a statement about the void in our knowledge about what is gained and lost by vertical integration and about why and how managers decide to integrate. This chapter contains a proposal for a research strategy to increase our knowledge. The health care sector provides a rich empirical crucible, and research on the theoretical debate could shed light on the problem of runaway costs in health care.

References

Balakrishnan, S., and Wernerfelt, B. "Technical Change, Competition and Vertical Integration." *Strategic Management Journal,* 1986, *7,* 347–359.

Barney, J. B., and Ouchi, W. E. (eds.). *Organizational Economics: Toward a New Paradigm for Understanding and Studying Organizations.* San Francisco: Jossey-Bass, 1986.

Blois, K. J. "Vertical Quasi-Integration." *Journal of Industrial Economy,* 1972, *20,* 253–272.

Clement, J. P. "Vertical Integration and Diversification of Acute Care Hospitals: Conceptual Definitions." *Hospital and Health Services Administration,* 1988, *33* (1), 99–110.

Conrad, D. A., Mick, S. S., Madden, C. W., and Hoare, G. "Vertical Structures and Control in Health Care Markets: A Conceptual Framework and Empirical Review." *Medical Care Review,* 1988, *45* (1), 49–100.

Cook, K. S. "Exchange and Power in Networks of Interorganizational Relations." *Sociological Quarterly,* 1977, *18,* 62–82.

Cyert, R. M., and March, J. G. *A Behavioral Theory of the Firm.* Englewood Cliffs, N.J.: Prentice-Hall, 1963.

Dess, G. G., and Beard, D. W. "Dimensions of Organizational Task Environments." *Administrative Science Quarterly,* 1984, *29* (1), 52–73.

Eccles, R. G. *The Transfer Pricing Problem: A Theory for Practice.* Lexington, Mass.: Lexington Books, 1985.

Emery, F. E., and Trist, E. L. "The Causal Texture of Organizational Environments." *Human Relations,* 1965, *18,* 21–32.

Evan, W. M. (ed.). *Interorganizational Relations.* Philadelphia: University of Pennsylvania Press, 1978.

Francis, A., Turk, J., and William, P. (eds.). *Power, Efficiency and Institutions: A Critical Appraisal of the "Markets and Hierarchies" Paradigm.* London: Heinemann, 1983.

Granovetter, M. "Economic Action and Social Structure: The Problem of Embeddedness." *American Journal of Sociology,* 1985, *91* (3), 481-510.

Griffith, J. R. *The Well-Managed Community Hospital.* Ann Arbor, Mich: Health Administration Press, 1987.

Hannan, M. T., and Freeman, J. *Organizational Ecology.* Cambridge, Mass.: Harvard University Press, 1989.

Harrigan, K. R. *Strategies for Vertical Integration.* Lexington, Mass.: Lexington Books, 1983.

Harrigan, K. R. "Formulating Vertical Integration Strategies." *Academy of Management Review,* 1984, *9* (4), 638-652.

Harrigan, K. R. *Strategic Flexibility: A Management Guide for Changing Times.* Lexington, Mass.: Lexington Books, 1985a.

Harrigan, K. R. "Vertical Integration and Corporate Strategy." *Academy of Management Journal,* 1985b, *28,* 397-425.

Jacobson, C. K. "A Conceptual Framework for Evaluating Joint Venture Opportunities Between Hospitals and Physicians." *Health Services Management Research,* 1989, *2* (3), 204-212.

Jauch, L. R., and Kraft, K. L. "Strategic Management of Uncertainty." *Academy of Management Review,* 1986, *11* (4), 777-790.

Karpik, L. (ed.). *Organization and Environment: Theory, Issues and Reality.* Beverly Hills, Calif.: Sage, 1978.

Mick, S. S., and Conrad, D. A. "The Decision to Integrate Vertically in Health Care Organizations." *Journal of Hospital and Health Services Administration,* 1988, *33,* 345-360.

Milliken, F. J. "Three Types of Perceived Uncertainty About the Environment: State, Effect, and Response Uncertainty." *Academy of Management Review,* 1987, *12* (1), 133-143.

Moe, T. M. "The New Economics of Organization." *American Journal of Political Science,* 1984, *28* (4), 739-777.

Ouchi, W. G. "Review of Markets and Hierarchies." *Administrative Science Quarterly,* 1977, *22,* 541-544.

Perrow, C. "Markets, Hierarchies and Hegemony." In A. H. Van de Ven and W. F. Joyce (eds.), *Perspectives on Organization Design and Behavior.* New York: Wiley, 1981.

Perrow, C. *Complex Organizations: A Critical Essay.* (3rd ed.) New York: Random House, 1986.

Pfeffer, J., and Salancik, G. R. *The External Control of Organiza-*

tions: A Resource Dependence Perspective. New York: Harper & Row, 1978.

Porter, M. E. *Competitive Strategy: Techniques for Analyzing Industries and Competitors.* New York: Free Press, 1980.

Robins, J. A. *Competitive Advantage: Creating and Sustaining Superior Performance.* New York: Free Press, 1985.

————. "Organizational Economics: Notes on the Use of Transaction-Cost Theory in the Study of Organizations." *Administrative Science Quarterly,* 1987, *32* (1), 68–86.

Simon, H. A. *Models of Man.* New York: Wiley, 1957.

Starbuck, W. H. "Organizations and Their Environments." In M. D. Dunnette (ed.), *Handbook of Industrial and Organizational Psychology.* Chicago: Rand McNally, 1976.

Stevens, R. *In Sickness and Wealth: American Hospitals in the Twentieth Century.* New York: Basic Books, 1989.

Thompson, J. D. *Organizations in Action.* New York: McGraw-Hill, 1967.

Walker, G., and Weber, D. "A Transaction Cost Approach to Make-or-Buy Decisions." *Administrative Science Quarterly,* 1984, *29,* 373–391.

Williamson, O. E. "The Vertical Integration of Production: Market Failure Considerations." *American Economic Review,* 1971, *61,* 112–123.

————. *Markets and Hierarchies: Analysis and Antitrust Implications.* New York: Free Press, 1975.

————. *The Economic Institutions of Capitalism.* New York: Free Press, 1985.

Williamson, O. E., and Ouchi, W. G. "A Rejoinder." In A. H. Van de Ven and W. F. Joyce (eds.), *Perspectives on Organization Design and Behavior.* New York: Wiley, 1981.

9

Managed-Care Systems
as Governance Structures:
A Transaction-Cost
Interpretation

Robert E. Hurley
Mary L. Fennell

Case management has become an extensively used though widely
varied approach to restructuring health-service delivery systems in
the United States. In a case-management, or managed-care, system,
a designated provider or broker of services assumes a contractual
responsibility to assure that a program beneficiary is able to obtain
appropriate health services on a timely basis. Despite the pervasiveness of both the language and apparatus of case management, the
concept remains loosely specified and weakly anchored in social
science and, especially, organization theory. These shortcomings in
turn have a direct influence on attempts to assess and evaluate how
case-managed delivery systems may be desirable alternatives to "un-
managed" delivery systems.

Case-management programs may be interpreted as emerging
from failure—market failure. We develop here a market-failure
perspective in the context of an analytical framework called
transaction-cost economics; this perspective has been applied only
recently to the analysis of health-service organizations. We portray
managed-care systems as efforts by purchasers to obtain health care
in an efficient and effective manner, and we interpret the systems
as a strategy to compensate for the fact that reliance on the invisible

hand of the marketplace does not result in minimizing the costs of care. As a rudimentary structure to govern health care transactions, case management theoretically may lead to improved administrative control and rationality in the acquisition of health services. There have been few empirical attempts to test that assumption or to develop a keen sense of under what conditions it can be expected to hold.

We examine here, in general terms, models of case-management systems. We then introduce the transaction-cost framework and link it to the features of managed-care systems. We develop two illustrations of specific case-management programs to explore and demonstrate the applicability of the framework. Finally, we present a set of propositions that suggest specific areas toward which empirical analysis may be directed. In conclusion, we offer some observations regarding the ability of this line of inquiry to advance the use of transaction-cost economics in organization-theory research.

Managed-Care Systems

The origins of case management in the social services realm can be found in the 1960s (Austin, 1985). Applications in traditional health services are more recent and appear to be growing. These programs extend case management to such groups as Medicaid beneficiaries (Freund and Hurley, 1987), old people (Capitman, Hoskins, and Bernstein, 1986), people with disabilities (Wool, Guadagnoli, Thomas, and Mor, 1989), high-risk pregnant women (New York State Department of Health, 1988), AIDS patients (Knickman, 1987), exceptionally high-cost users (Henderson and Wallack, 1987), and people who are chronically mentally ill (Franklin and others, 1987). This wide assortment of programs and program models, with corresponding wide variations in program goals, has contributed to serious definitional and taxonomic problems in the study of case management.

A further difficulty in examining these programs is that what they appear to do depends on the vantage point or perspective from which one chooses to examine them. For the patient or beneficiary, a program may be markedly different from traditional delivery systems, while the providers of the service may find their modus oper-andi little altered. In other instances, the opposite case may be ob-served. Furthermore, some of these programs impose on delivery systems third-party brokers or intermediaries who may be viewed as either facilitators or intruders, again depending on the observer's vantage point.

In addition to the perspectives of the beneficiary and the providers, we will also be discussing that of the purchaser. This perspective is chosen because purchasers currently provide the prin-cipal impetus for cost-containment initiatives after passively bear-ing the brunt of enormous increases in health care costs for several decades. Purchasers are either contractually or legislatively obli-gated to acquire for beneficiaries prespecified packages of benefits. Assuming economic prudence on the part of purchasers, one ex-pects them to be motivated by the desire to obtain benefits in the most cost-effective manner possible. Furthermore, one can expect purchasers to adapt their buying strategies to take into account the particular characteristics of the goods and services being produced and of the transactions through which these goods and services are acquired.

We will argue here that case-management strategies have been adopted because purchasers of health services have concluded that allowing beneficiaries to acquire services individually in the market-place via so-called spot-market purchases is inappropriate or ineffi-cient for many health-service transactions. Contrary to the notions of the perfectly competitive marketplace, entering and reentering the marketplace for each discrete purchase (spot-market purchasing) is simply not cost effective. In other words, the imperfections or fail-ures of certain markets propel purchasers to use other mechanisms to assure a stable supply of needed services. Through these mecha-nisms, they attempt to remove from the marketplace those transac-tions that can be efficiently carried out by using prearranged governance structures—sustained contractual relationships with providers or service brokers or both. The expected net effect of these arrangements is the reduction of the transaction costs of arranging services. Because transaction costs are added to provider production costs to determine total acquisition costs, one can see why purchasers are interested in reducing transaction costs.

Merrill (1985) proposes a simple but useful set of three models of case management that appear to accommodate the current spectrum of programs: medical, sociomedical, and social. These models include both the nature of beneficiary services to be case managed and the requisite expertise of the case manager. We briefly describe each of these models here.

Medical case-management programs focus on the recruitment of medical providers (physicians) who assume responsibility to provide or authorize (or both) a specified range of medical services to beneficiaries who are formally enrolled with the provider. Characteristically, enrollees relinquish their choice of provider after selecting a case manager. The case manager becomes the gatekeeper, the enrollees' sole point of initial access to services (Freund, 1984). Case managers, by virtue of being medical professionals and having most medical services within their purview of responsibility, are expected to exercise professional discretion in their decision making about the type and extent of medical care required by their beneficiaries.

These programs typically have two key purposes. One is to assure beneficiary access to a stable, certain supply of medical care; the other is to impose some regimentation on the utilization patterns of these beneficiaries. Regimentation, especially exemplified in the Medicaid program, which has extensively employed medical case management, is anchored in the expectation that the costs of acquiring care can be contained or reduced by judicious gatekeeping, or provider-managed access to care. For example, primary-care gatekeeping is viewed as having the potential to reduce the use of unneeded services; to shift care from inappropriate (more costly) sites such as emergency departments and specialist physicians; and to limit the inefficiencies associated with "doctor shopping" (Freund, 1984). To increase the likelihood of these effects, purchasers like Medicaid commonly use various financial incentives for primary-care case managers.

Sociomedical case-management programs are designed to manage the delivery of services to persons who are in actual or potential need of a combination of both medical and social services, which may be either service complements or substitutes. Persons with chronic medical conditions or who face an intensive regimen of treatment for which alternative modes exist may have the delivery of their care managed. Considerable variation in the qualifications of sociomedical case managers may be noted. In some instances, medical professionals, including nurses as well as physicians, may perform this role, while in others the position may be a more purely brokering one, carried out by community-services or health workers such as social workers. Brokers play both advisory and advocacy roles in their identification and arrangement of services on behalf of beneficiaries. Case management for those who are chronically mentally ill is an example of this model.

Purchasers exhibit interest in this sociomedical model for both access and cost-containment reasons and also for the apparent benefits in coordination that may be derived from having one person oversee all service delivery. Because of the potential for substituting less costly and, perhaps, more appropriate modes of supportive and treatment services, the argument for a case manager of this type can be quite compelling for certain conditions. In addition, for persons who need multiple and diverse services, overlapping and disjointed service-delivery networks may be confusing, disruptive, and inefficient. Thus, the case manager may be expected to assist in negotiating and coordinating service delivery in such cases.

In contrast to the role of the medical case manager, the role of the sociomedical case manager is not necessarily already being performed by a traditional professional; for example, a primary-care physican may be viewed as an implicit case manager or gatekeeper for his or her patients (Berenson, 1985). However, the sociomedical case manager is typically imposed by the purchaser because of the belief that a coordinator or broker with sufficient clinical expertise and knowledge of the service-delivery system can assure the delivery of a superior product to the beneficiary. This issue is addressed further in the mental health case-management illustration later in the chapter.

In addition to medical and sociomedical models, Merrill (1985) proposes the model of social case management. The focus in this model is primarily, if not exclusively, on the coordinating or brokering function. Because this model applies solely to social services rather than health services and because social-service personnel are the usual case managers, it is distinct in important ways from the two previous case-management models. The model is of interest here, however, primarily because it illustrates that purchasers of social services apparently believe that imposition of a case manager can provide beneficiaries with advocacy, information, and referral assistance, without which purchaser acquisition of services would be less efficient and effective.

In summary, the potential benefits of adopting case management may be substantial for health-service purchasers. These benefits would seem, however, to be contingent on buyers' carefully selecting those kinds of services for which managed care is a desirable alternative to spot-market acquisition. It is necessary then to identify the types of transactions for which case management or a governance structure is the preferred method of transacting with suppliers.

Transaction-Cost Economics

Williamson's work on the theory of transaction-cost economics (1975, 1981, 1986) provides a framework within which case management can be analyzed. Most fundamentally, Williamson has developed an approach to "dimensionalizing" transactions to identify those for which discrete market purchases are considered inferior to long-term relational contracting. After first elaborating this framework, we will explore the dimensions of medical care transactions to illustrate which types are most suited for governance via case management. Following this general treatment, two specific types of case-management programs will be examined to assess their fit with this theoretical model.

Theoretical Framework. Williamson (1975) argues that organizations (governance structures or "hierarchies") emerge as a consequence of market failure. Where the marketplace fails to provide the most efficient mode of exchange for goods or services, governance structures arise to permit buyers to minimize the transaction costs associated with exchanges with suppliers. The organizing principle is the minimization of the sum of transaction and production costs, and the "efficient boundaries" of organizations result from the quest to achieve this minimization. In Williamson's (1986) terms a governance structure is an institutional matrix within which transactions can be negotiated and executed.

The unit of analysis in this approach is the transaction. Williamson suggests that optimal contractual relationships among buyers and suppliers are dictated by the characteristics of their transactions. Many transactions are well served by spot-market exchange, in which purchasers and suppliers have little or no continuing contractual obligations. Other transactions are less suited for such simple exchange because of informational asymmetries (Arrow, 1963) or other complicating factors. In extreme cases, removing the transactions from the market altogether and organizing internally (vertical integration) may be the most suitable approach to minimizing transaction costs.

Dimensions. Williamson (1986) describes three critical dimensions of transactions: uncertainty, frequency, and identity or interchangeability of suppliers. Uncertainty is a pervasive and unavoidable problem that purchasers face when promising beneficiaries services on demand for medical problems. If we assume that uncertainty of future service needs is a given (Williamson, 1986), the frequency and identity dimensions become key differentiators with which to analyze transactions. As shown in Figure 9.1, the frequency of transactions may be classified as occasional and recurrent and the importance of supplier identity (investment characteristics) may be arrayed from nonspecific (or interchangeable) to mixed to idiosyncratic (or where the identity of the supplier matters).

When transactions are frequent and suppliers are interchangeable, market governance is adequate to assure that costs of arranging services are minimized. The specific identity of the supplier is irrelevant as each purchase is discrete and there are no transaction costs associated with buying from different suppliers each time. Alternatively, frequent transactions that must be concentrated with a single supplier whose identity is important invariably have high transaction costs if market governance is relied on. Because of specialized physical-capital needs or human-capital investment ("asset specificity"), the suppliers are no longer interchangeable, and thus buyers' prerogatives are constrained. As a result, a sustained relationship provides an opportunity to reduce purchaser

Figure 9.1. Dimensions of Transactions.

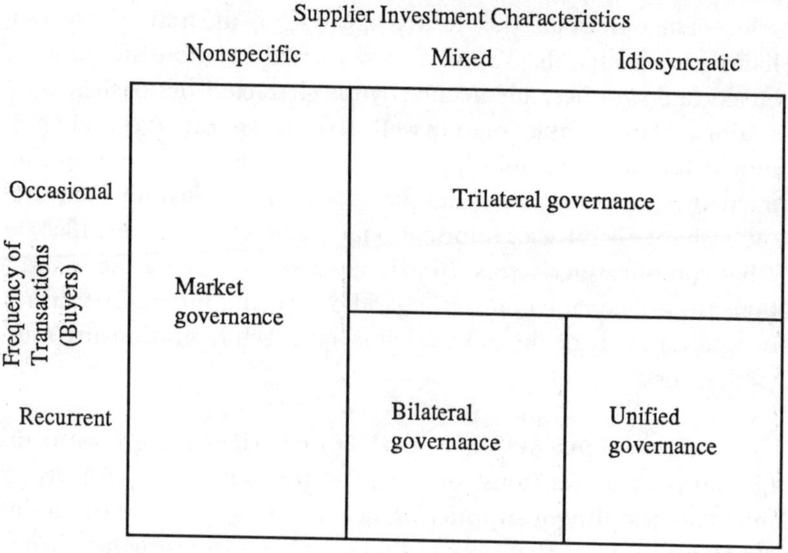

Supplier Investment Characteristics

	Nonspecific	Mixed	Idiosyncratic

Occasional		Trilateral governance
Market governance		
Recurrent	Bilateral governance	Unified governance

Frequency of Transactions (Buyers)

vulnerability to opportunistic behavior by suppliers, which raises transaction costs. In the extreme case, a unified governance structure may be deemed most well suited. This process of deciding on the best governance structure is less formally known as performing make-or-buy decisions, which, in Williamson's (1981) terms, ultimately produce the efficient boundaries of a firm (also, Walker and Weber, 1984).

Figure 9.1 illustrates a complete set of the governance structures that Williamson (1986) suggests are the preferred modes for minimizing transaction costs. Market governance suffices when suppliers are interchangeable. For occasional transactions where supplier identity has an impact on transaction costs, a long-term contractual relationship can suffice, but a third party may be necessary to resolve disputes by acting as an arbitrator (trilateral contracting). In recurrent or frequent transactions when the specific identity of the supplier influences transaction costs, bilateral governance (relational contracting) or a unified governance arrangement is desirable.

Transaction-cost economics has a number of other useful

components as elaborated by Williamson (1986). Several of these features pertain to the benefits of relational contracting and unified governance structures. Stable, sustained relationships permit tight monitoring or metering of the performance of suppliers by purchasers. This information can then be used to calculate "experience ratings" of suppliers, including assessment of compliance with contractual guarantees or, in worst cases, grounds for contract termination. In the unified governance arrangement, this process becomes, in essence, a performance appraisal for employees. Another feature of relational contracts and especially unified governance structures is that divergent economic motives can be subordinated to a joint profit-maximization goal, thereby reducing the likelihood of conflict and competitive behavior. This framework may be used to examine case management as a governance structure to minimize transaction costs.

Case Management as Rudimentary Governance Structure

Third-party purchasers are faced with health care markets notorious for their imperfections and their failures (Arrow, 1963). In their search for mechanisms that will enable them to purchase prudently and effectively for their beneficiaries, they have adopted case management in a number of instances, presumably because of the belief that it can compensate for these imperfections and failures. In Williamson's terminology, case management is a buyer approach to minimizing transaction costs when market governance is not the preferred mode of exchange with certain suppliers.

A critical step in exploring how case management fits into the transaction-cost framework is to attempt to dimensionalize medical care transactions by frequency and interchangeability of suppliers and to ascertain the exchange mechanisms that appear most suitable for different classes of these transactions. Figure 9.2 is a simplified attempt to make these judgments. The frequency-of-transactions dimension is self-explanatory; placement on this dimension is determined largely by the prevalence of the conditions necessitating service use. The supplier-identity dimension is of greater interest and importance than the frequency dimension and requires further development.

Figure 9.2. Dimensions of Medical Transactions.

Supplier Investment Characteristics

	Nonspecific	Mixed	Idiosyncratic
Occasional	Optician	Exotic specialties	Hospital
Recurrent	Pharmacy	Common specialties	Primary care

Frequency of Transactions (Buyers)

The purchase of such services or commodities as eyeglasses or prescription drugs may be achieved via open-market transactions because the identity of the suppliers of these goods has relatively little importance and thus little or no impact on transaction costs. In the middle or mixed range, the identity of the suppliers or providers has some importance because there is merit in having a sustained relationship to guarantee reliability and accountability of performance. Specialist physicians of both the exotic (subspecialists) and common varieties typically see patients on referral from other physicians with whom they maintain continuing exchange relationships. Interestingly, then, the purchaser relationship with these suppliers is typically mediated by the primary-care provider. In a similar vein, the hospital relationship is mediated through the admitting physician. Thus, the admitting primary-care physician in effect functions like a third-party arbitrator in what Williamson has characterized as "trilateral contracting," as shown in Figure 9.1.

The final cell in Figure 9.2 is a critical position, occupied by the supplier of primary care who provides recurrent care and whose identity clearly matters. This supplier has, in Williamson's terms, "asset specificity" owing to relationships with the beneficiary and with the other suppliers engaged in medical-care transactions with the purchaser. Through getting to know the beneficiaries and their medical histories and maintaining pertinent clinical data in individual medical records, the primary-care physician obtains valuable information that can be used to both the patient's and the physician's advantage. This asymmetry of information possession places the purchaser in a potentially disadvantaged position with respect to the minimization of transaction costs. Furthermore, as clinical gatekeeper to referral sources like specialists and hospitals, the primary-care physician possesses significant influence on production as well as transaction costs.

The basic challenge for the purchaser is to engage this supplier in a relationship that minimizes susceptibility to opportunistic behavior and increases the likelihood that joint profit-maximizing behavior will occur. A case-management model, in this instance primary-care case management, may afford an opportunity to achieve these goals. By formally enrolling beneficiaries with designated primary-care case managers and thereafter restricting freedom of choice, the purchaser is exploiting the pivotal role the primary-care physician plays in making resource-allocation decisions. Judicious use of financial incentives, such as shared savings from reduced referral care, may curb opportunistic behavior and align the physician's goals with those of the purchaser. In addition, the general structure of enrollment permits the desired tight metering and experience rating of the performance of primary-care physicians.

In effect, a primary-care case-management system creates a rudimentary governance structure. The organizing principle for this structure is the potential for economizing on transaction costs through the special relationship that primary-care physicians have with their patients. To assess the impact of the structure on transaction costs it is necessary to distinguish between production and transaction costs. Production costs are those costs incurred by providers of medical care in producing services that contribute to the optimal health status of a beneficiary. Transaction costs are expenses associated with searching, arranging, coordinating, and contracting; they are incurred by the purchaser of services seeking to assure the availability of a predetermined package of benefits. This distinction is discussed further following our presentation of illustrative managed-care systems.

Illustrations of Case Management

To explore this general transaction-cost interpretation of case management, we examine two different case-management programs. The first of these is a medical case-management model and the second is a medicosocial case-management approach. The examinations address the goals these programs attempt to achieve and the operational designs they adopt. We present selected empirical evidence of program effects in order to assess whether these findings are consistent with expectations arising from the transaction-cost framework.

Primary-Care Case Management in Medicaid. More than thirty state Medicaid agencies have developed some form of primary-care case-management programs since 1981, when changes in federal requirements began to permit and encourage the proliferation of this strategy (Freund and Neuschler, 1986). An extensive descriptive literature is available on these programs, in which Medicaid agencies engage a subset of all Medicaid providers to become primary-care case managers (Hurley, 1986). Eligible beneficiaries then select one of these case managers and relinquish their freedom to choose other providers. Virtually all medical care for the beneficiaries must be provided or authorized by the case manager with whom they have enrolled. Most of these programs have been mandatory for beneficiaries in certain eligibility categories. A few have been voluntary—beneficiaries retain the option of remaining in the traditional Medicaid program, which continues to run parallel to the case-managed system (Prottas and Handler, 1987).

The principal goals of Medicaid agencies for primary-care case management have been cost containment and assurance of beneficiary access to necessary care (Freund and Hurley, 1987). The strategy is viewed as a potential solution to the persistent Medicaid problems of unnecessary care, constrained access to primary-care providers (which results in services in inappropriate and excessively costly sites) and inefficiencies and discontinuities in care seeking because of freedom of choice, including self-referral to specialists. Channeling beneficiary access through a primary-care case manager can, in theory, address many of these problems because, in the terms of transaction-cost economics, the primary-care physician has asset specificity, and thus a governance structure such as case management would be the preferred mode of exchange. Moreover, the use of financial incentives including capitation (fixed prepayments based on expected rather than actual use), case-manager fees, and shared savings opportunities may be expected to increase the effectiveness with which the primary-care doctor performs case-management functions. Such incentives may also be viewed as attempts to curb provider opportunism by aligning potential gains for the physician with those of the purchaser (in this case, the Medicaid agency).

A substantial base of empirical evidence has been accumulated from more than fifteen of these Medicaid primary-care case-management programs (Freund and others, 1988; Adler, Holahan, and Bell, 1987; McCall and others, 1988; Davidson and others, 1988). These findings can be examined to assess how patterns of care seeking and provision may have been altered in these purchaser-inspired alternative delivery systems. Of special interest is whether the evidence suggests that primary-care case management is reducing the transaction costs incurred by the Medicaid agency.

Several noteworthy effects on beneficiary use patterns have been reported. These programs have consistently found sharp reductions in the use of the emergency department as a source of primary care (Hurley, Freund, and Taylor, 1989). By eliminating this care or diverting it to a primary-care physician's office, Medicaid avoids the increased expense of using this site. Enrollees in primary-care case-management programs also are less likely than those who are not in managed programs to see a medical specialist and to receive ancillary services and commodities like laboratory tests, X-rays, and prescription drugs (Freund and others, 1988). In addition, the enrollees receive their services from fewer providers than do similar persons remaining in the traditional Medicaid program. Evidence with respect to reductions in inpatient stays are more mixed, probably because there is relatively little discretionary (elective) inpatient use in this population. When financial incentives are used to intensify pressures on primary-care gatekeepers, some of these effects, like reductions in visits to specialists and in inpatient care are amplified.

These effects are broadly consistent with expectations of the program design. They may also be interpreted as evidence that Medicaid's transaction costs are being reduced. For example, care diverted from the emergency department or the specialist's office to a primary-care physician reduces expenditures while providing, presumably, a clinically equivalent product (maintaining, restoring, or improving health). The reductions in ancillary use are consistent with reductions in the redundancies that result, for example, from patients going to multiple providers without access to prior test results. Reducing the number of providers treating beneficiaries decreases the discontinuities of care and the excessive use of ancillary services that arise in a freedom-of-choice environment. Moreover, this increased concentration may explain why little evidence of increased primary-care visits to offset specialist and emergency-room reductions has been found (Hurley, Freund, and Taylor, 1989).

In sum, the evidence reviewed indicates that primary-care case management can produce a number of effects on patterns of service acquisition. These effects are consistent with and supportive of a transaction-cost minimization strategy embraced by a purchaser that has adopted medical case management as a governance structure. It is interesting, however, that overall savings from these programs have generally been viewed by Medicaid officials as relatively marginal, ranging from 0 to 15 percent depending on the particular program designs. Those programs with financial incentives have consistently shown larger savings than those without them. Although official disappointment is probably a consequence of unreasonable expectations, the sources and amount of savings suggest that it may be transaction costs, not production costs, that are reduced by the use of primary-care case management. None of the studies cited explicitly attempted to investigate the distinction between transaction and production costs or cost savings.

Case Management in the Delivery of Mental Health Services. The concept of case management became increasingly popular in the mental health sector in the 1980s. However, the extent of its diffusion was erratic, and no standard definition of case management has been uniformly accepted. In general, case management in mental health has strongly emphasized the broker, or coordinating, role of the sociomedical model, and this emphasis is nowhere more clearly suggested than in the analysis of case management for those who are chronically mentally ill and those who are homeless and mentally ill. Service coordination and, more recently, client advocacy have been described as necessary functions performed by mental health case managers to increase access to the wide variety of mental health, medical, and social welfare services needed by those who are seriously mentally ill.

The prominence of the service-coordinator role can be understood given the history of the delivery of mental health services since deinstitutionalization. Although the community mental health center was intended to replace the centralized state mental hospital as the cornerstone of mental health delivery, in fact what developed was a complex, fragmented, decentralized array of service providers (Levine and Fleming, 1986). Community mental health centers were by and large unprepared to serve chronic mental patients and those without stable living arrangements (Bassuk, 1986; Mechanic, 1986). Case management moved to fill the void and has emerged as a key factor in charting long-term courses of therapy and rehabilitation for people who are chronically mentally ill, most of whom require assistance in obtaining both mental health and medical services, the benefits of entitlement programs, housing, rehabilitation for alcohol and drug abuse, and other social welfare services.

As described by Levine and Fleming (1986), the National Institute of Mental Health (NIMH) has been involved in assisting states in their development of "community support systems" since the early 1970s: "The NIMH definition of a community support system includes a service integration function, or case management function, as one of its ten essential services" (p. 4). In more recent policy plans, integrative services have been identified as one of the basic needs of those who are chronically mentally ill (Department of Health and Human Services, 1981), and others have equated the integration function with case management (Schwartz, Goldman, and Churgin, 1982; Intagliata, 1982; Levine and Fleming, 1986):

"Recently, case management has been viewed as the primary and perhaps essential means for assuring that an adequate and appropriate range of services are provided to mentally disabled individuals who are now residing in communities . . . to make more efficient use of the existing network of human services" (Levine and Fleming, 1986, p. 7).

This emphasis on the efficient use of services would qualify mental health case management as the type of governance structure one would predict from transaction-cost analysis. However, formally sanctioned program goals and operational designs of case-management programs are less obviously reflective of the desire to reduce costs than they are of the need to assure client access to services.

To examine the transactions necessary in acquiring mental health services, the framework of Figure 9.1 is again useful. As before, the frequency of transactions is quite important, and we should distinguish between clients who are in need of recurrent service delivery (seriously mentally ill patients, chronic mental patients) and those who are perhaps episodically in need of counseling or short-term therapy. The investment characteristics may be conceptualized simply as a relational dichotomy: nonspecific or idiosyncratic. In transactions in mental health services, the identity of the supplier or provider is of special importance, at least for the duration of a particular therapeutic regimen. However, the supplier's asset specificity is less important if the client's illness is simple and requires a fairly standard period and type of therapy than if the client's condition is complex and requires multiple therapies, sequencing of interventions, and coordination of multiple service providers. Asset specificity in such transactions is based on the service provider's special knowledge of the client's diverse needs, history, and long-term treatment plan, as well as knowledge of other providers and services needed in the course of treatment (see Figure 9.3).

Within this framework, case management may be interpreted as a desirable governance structure for transactions involving those who are chronically mentally ill and others in need of long-term, complex treatment. Short-term, simple counseling or therapy, of the sort often sought by relatively affluent, well-educated clients,

Figure 9.3. Dimensions of Mental Health Transactions.

Supplier Investment Characteristics

	Nonspecific	Idiosyncratic
Occasional	Short-term counseling for adjustment disorders	Family crisis intervention
Recurrent	Alcoholics Anonymous	Long-term treatment or rehabilitation for chronic mental illness

Frequency of Transactions (Buyers)

can be efficiently transacted through the mental health system's version of the spot market: personal referral or recommendation of local practitioners in private practice.

A review of selected state and local case-management programs (Rog, Andranovich, and Rosenblum, 1987) reports that most programs at both levels tend to focus on six basic goals: client identification and outreach; assessment of client needs, strengths, and deficits; development of comprehensive service plans; linkage with necessary services; monitoring of service delivery; and client advocacy. Unlike the situation in the primary-care case-management example, cost containment is usually not an explicit goal, although the emphasis on monitoring of service delivery could be viewed as an indirect approach to cost reduction, secondary to the overriding objective of meeting clients' needs. As Levine and Fleming argue (1986): "The objectives of the monitoring function are to assure that the client is receiving the expected services and that these services are necessary and appropriate for the client" (p. 14). Of course, if managed care resulted in the delivery of only needed services, at the most appropriate time, and in the most efficient manner, transaction costs would be lowered.

Another major difference in emphasis between the primary-care example and mental health case management is the central importance in mental health of case finding. Case managers can identify clients who need mental health services but who might otherwise have no system contact, and they thereby increase the access of such difficult-to-reach clients to the full range of services they might need to improve their health status. Client advocacy and client outreach in mental health case management emphasize the importance of locating those who are chronically mentally ill and in so doing underscore the extent to which such clients either are not cognizant of how to find the various services and systems they need or, in many cases, are in fact not cognizant that they are in need of such services. With case management the responsibility for performing these functions can be lodged with a contractually obligated case manager and performance can be monitored systematically.

As a group, the chronically mentally ill are not ordinarily able to engage effectively in spot-market transactions of any sort, and thus purchasers of care for them are exposed to opportunistic or at least misguided behavior on the part of providers and practitioners in various service systems, such as hospital emergency departments or the police. Often a homeless person who is chronically mentally ill will surface in a holding cell, detoxification center, or emergency psychiatric ward for treatment of an acute crisis and then be released again to the streets until the next episode. Through outreach efforts to locate such clients and engage them in a sustained, case-managed program of coordinated services, it may be possible to decrease the probability of the crisis episode and of inappropriate or costly (or both) responses to it.

Obviously, increasing the system's total caseload could lead to increased total acquisition costs. However, some of these cost increases may be offset by the lowered transaction costs realized through eliminating or reducing both redundancy and the discontinuity in care that occur when clients attempt to self-refer to inappropriate agencies. Cost increases may also be offset through ultimately lowered societal costs obtained by decreasing the number of mentally ill street people entering the system through contacts with police (Dockett, 1986) and by increasing the overall size and productivity of the labor force through job rehabilitation.

Case management in mental health differs from the primary-care example not only in goals but also in operational designs. In mental health case management there may be no traditional professional or de facto broker or intermediary to assume the case-manager role. Rather, the literature on mental health case mangement suggests that case-manager job descriptions can (and should) be discipline-independent (Levine and Fleming, 1986) and that either individuals or teams can perform case-management functions. Whether mental health professionals, case-management specialists, paid staff, volunteers, or indigenous workers are used as case managers should depend on the type of service agency and the mix of resources available. Effective case management depends on the appropriate mix of personal attributes—"growth-oriented" attitudes toward clients (Gersten, 1981), the ability to tolerate ambiguity and long-term lack of results, bureaucratic "savvy"—knowledge of a number of treatment-related areas (management of chronic mental illness, psychotropic medications and side effects, community resources, rehabilitation, the legal system); and interpersonal skills related to interviewing, teaching, assessing needs (Levine and Fleming, 1986).

There has been considerable discussion concerning whether mental health professionals, especially clinicians or therapists, should take on the case-management role, or whether case management should be a freestanding, specially designated program. Using professionals as case managers runs the risk of relying inappropriately on traditional therapeutic strategies rather than emphasizing service coordination and links to other providers. Thus, the coordination goals of case management could be jeopardized (Levine and Fleming, 1986; Rog, Andranovich, and Rosenblum, 1987). Alternatively, the establishment of a separate case-management program or agency could itself be prohibitively expensive, thus canceling out expected transaction-cost savings.

Another dimension on which case management within the mental health system can vary is the manner and the extent to which case managers are authorized or empowered to exercise authority.

Levine and Fleming (1986) outline several alternative ap-

proaches. The most common is to rely on mental health professionals as case managers, in which case the authority of the expert is
expected to carry over. Another strategy is for either the state or local
mental health authority to explicitly designate a specific agency as
the legitimate portal of entry into the mental health delivery system,
in which case only that agency's case managers would have the
authority to refer clients to specific services (Intagliata, 1982). A
related strategy is to vest case managers with purchase-of-service
power. In this case they both refer clients for service and provide
payment for services rendered, thereby encouraging substitution of
less costly services. Finally, case-manager authority can be officially
enhanced through the use of formal policy agreements or legislative
mandates or both (Schwartz, Goldman, and Churgin, 1982). The
choice of alternative approaches varies depending on the goals of
program sponsors and the types of transaction costs they are most
intent on reducing.

   Although several studies have shown positive cost-benefit results from case management in mental health delivery (Mueller and
Hopp, 1983; Wasylenki and others, 1985; Perlman, Melnick, and
Kentera, 1985), few of these studies were able to measure directly the
extent to which transaction-cost reductions occurred. The Mueller
and Hopp study found a reduction in frequency and duration of
rehospitalization following case management for discharged mental
patients, although utilization of community resources and services
did not increase. The Perlman, Melnick, and Kentera study found
that case management within a community support system in
Yonkers (New York) was effective in linking clients to psychosocial
services, but there was no control comparison.

   Whether transaction costs actually decline as a result of case
management in mental health needs considerable additional study.
At least two environmental factors may have an important influence
on achieving such cost reductions: the extent to which the community actually provides an adequate supply of needed services for
those who are severely mentally ill, and the extent to which interagency relations allow for effective service links and client referrals.
Levine and Fleming argue (1986) that when services for those who
are chronically mentally ill are in general available and accessible,
the case manager can indeed function as a "traffic officer" (p. 36;

see also Beatrice, 1979, p. 19) to reduce service duplication and unnecessary referrals. However, where services are scarce, the case manager is likely to spend a good deal of time either attempting to provide services (therapy, counseling) directly to clients to make up for the gaps in service availability or to refer clients to a costly provider for lack of alternatives. In the case of referrals, a reduction in transaction costs would be unlikely or at least difficult to estimate because of the inadequate service base.

The effectiveness of case managers in achieving transaction-cost reductions may also be adversely affected where interagency relations are hostile or where domain conflicts preclude cooperative referrals. Blocked referrals and the unwillingness of some agencies to accept some client (especially those who are chronically ill or those who are homeless and mentally ill) may preclude case managers from maximizing the use of appropriate, and least costly, providers. The strength of such blocks depends on the type or combination (or both) of authorization strategies chosen to legitimate case-manager referrals and on expectations of service delivery and follow-up. If these obstacles cannot be overcome, spot-market acquisition becomes the default strategy for purchasers.

Research Guided by Transaction-Cost Economics

These two illustrations argue for the potential utility of employing a transaction-cost framework in case-management research. The following discussion develops a series of propositions regarding case management that may be adapted to formulate testable hypotheses in the specific contexts of a variety of case-management programs and models.

Limitations on entry into medical care systems may be expected to suppress the number of service contacts a beneficiary has, especially if system resources have been abundant and some of the contacts have been nonessential. Moreover, case managers possess asset specificity either because of the nature of the services they supply or because they have been appointed to the broker position by a purchaser. In performance of their delivery or arranging functions (or both), they accumulate important information about beneficiary needs and experiences that may allow them to avoid incurring start-up or other learning costs. Therefore, our first pro-position is that under conditions of resource abundance adoption of case management can lead to decreased levels of service duplica-tion and to reductions in redundant services provided to individual beneficiaries.

Purchasers may be vulnerable to opportunistic behavior by suppliers who possess information that may grant them a superior negotiating position. Sustained contractual relationships and uni-fied governance systems can avoid this problem by incorporating specific mechanisms such as capitation or shared-savings arrange-ments. Capitation may reduce vulnerability to opportunism by eliminating the incentives to encourage overuse of services. In ad-dition, these arrangements can encourage suppliers to seek out less costly alternatives for providing clinically equivalent services. Thus, our second proposition argues that case-management systems with mechanisms to curb supplier opportunism will lead to higher use of less costly service alternatives when compared with both freedom-of-choice systems and case-management systems without such mechanisms.

In a freedom-of-choice of supplier environment, no single provider has a clearly identified responsibility for rendering or coor-dinating an optimal mix of services. Given this diffusion of respon-sibility and accountability, purchasers are unable to evaluate adequately the appropriateness and effectiveness of the contribu-tions of individual suppliers to beneficiary health status. A case-management model may allow for clearly assigned responsibility and for the establishment of accountability through monitoring and assessing supplier performance. Therefore, our third proposi-tion is that case-management systems will lead to increased pur-chaser discrimination in supplier selection because of the opportunity for tighter metering and experience rating of supplier performance than in freedom-of-choice systems.

In some case-management models, the ability of the case manager to render as well as broker services provides beneficiaries with a guarantee of access to service when needed. The professional discretion of the provider-broker determines the scope of services provided or arranged through referral to other service providers. The pure broker model requires the case manager to select from among candidate providers the most appropriate supplier of services given the needs of the beneficiary. We would then expect our fourth proposition to hold: Under conditions of service or resource scarcity, case-management systems are likely to use provider-brokers as case managers.

The case-manager position is empowered or otherwise strengthened by lodging with the case manager the capacity to make the delivery system responsive to the beneficiary's needs. Requiring patients to obtain the authorization of a case manager before contacting other service providers is a common approach to accomplishing this empowerment. In addition, granting case managers a role in determining the referral and payment arrangements to other providers can garner the attention and cooperation of these providers. Effective case managers would be expected to exploit this position of influence to the benefit of their clients. Our fifth proposition thus is that to the extent case-management systems are structured with either legally mandated authority or financial clout, they will be more likely to provide comparable or superior access to service than freedom-of-choice systems do.

Potential Contribution of Transaction-Cost Analysis

The transaction-cost perspective has not been employed extensively in empirical work in organization theory. The root cause of this underuse appears to be the difficulty in defining transaction costs and distinguishing them convincingly from production costs. Overcoming this problem is no simpler in health-services research than elsewhere. In fact, it is probably more difficult.

The arguments advanced earlier for using this perspective depend on an important assumption: From the purchaser's point of view the acquisition of medical and mental health services is intended to produce some optimal level of or improvement in health status. The costs incurred by providers in attempting to produce this optimal health status are production costs. The costs incurred by purchasers in searching out, arranging, coordinating, and assuring the availability of these services on behalf of their beneficiaries are transaction costs. These transaction costs cannot be eliminated, but they may be minimized. Their minimization enables an increased portion of purchaser expenditures to go toward production costs.

Although transaction and production costs are easy to define, in practice they are often hard to determine. Purchasers often are accused of having simplistic, unsophisticated notions about the health services they are intent on acquiring because they expect producers and suppliers to provide precise measures of production costs and service effectiveness. When producers are understandably reluctant to do so, purchasers view themselves as susceptible to opportunistic behavior that may unnecessarily drive up transaction costs. However, such uncertainty is a legitimate source of unavoidable search and negotiation costs.

Careful analysis of the nature of transactions can provide purchasers with important guidance and insight into how best to structure them to minimize trransaction costs. Some transaction costs are more obvious than others. For example, repetition of laboratory or x-ray work when a patient is referred simply because the patient's records are not readily available inflates transaction costs. There is no value added by the production of these additional services. Alternatively, a referral by a primary-care physician to an eye surgeon for cataract surgery unavoidably incurs additional transaction costs because the provision of the needed service requires the surgeon's expertise. If this referral relationship is well established and the patient correspondingly is processed for surgery expeditiously, transaction costs can be minimized.

However, a less obvious case is referral by a primary-care physician to a specialist for a confirmatory diagnosis of a relatively easily identified condition. A strict interpretation would suggest that if the additional information secured does not lead to improved health status, the referral has increased transaction rather than production costs. In other words, the referral was a superfluous transaction cost, at least from the perspective of the purchaser. Unfortunately, such gray, murky areas are relatively common in health services, as is uncertainty concerning the efficacy of many treatments. But they are becoming less common than they once were, and significant progress is likely in determining "true" production costs.

The potential contribution of the transaction-cost perspective is that it suggests that organizing and structuring delivery systems and introducing incentives to curb opportunistic provider and supplier behavior can minimize transaction costs. A "bigger bang for the buck" is at least theoretically possible if purchasers buy shrewdly by organizing and negotiating their contracts with aggressiveness and ingenuity. Examination of the dimensions of medical care transactions is of fundamental importance in this regard.

The entire field of health care is moving toward increased uniformity in product specification and increasingly valid and reliable information on the efficiency and efficacy of production processes. In addition, purchaser expectations for provider accountability on economic and quality criteria are rising. Increased variability in sources of services is also available. Taken together, these trends afford unprecedented opportunities to employ precepts from organization theory and management that have traditionally encountered staunch resistance in health care enterprises. Like their macrolevel analogs, vertically integrated health care systems, managed-care systems present a promising opportunity to bring administrative structure and rationality to the important task of delivering health services.

References

Adler, G., Holahan, J., and Bell, J. (eds.). *Medicaid Program Evaluation: Final Report.* Working Paper 9.2. Baltimore: Office of Research and Development, Health Care Financing Administration, Department of Health and Human Services, 1987.

Arrow, K. "Uncertainty and the Welfare Economics of Medical Care." *American Economic Review,* 1963, *53* (5), 941–973.

Austin, C. D. "Case Management in Long Term Care: Options and Opportunity." *Health and Social Work,* 1985, *8* (1), 16–30.

Bassuk, E. (ed.). *The Mental Health Needs of Homeless Persons.* New Directions for Mental Health Services, no. 30. San Francisco: Jossey-Bass, 1986.

Beatrice, D. "Case Management: A Policy Option for Long Term Care." Unpublished doctoral dissertation, Brandeis University, 1979.

Berenson, R. "A Physician's Perspective on Case Management." *Business and Health,* July/Aug. 1985, pp. 21–24.

Capitman, J., Haskins, B., and Bernstein, J. "Case Management Approaches in Coordinated Community Long-Term Care Demonstrations." *The Gerontologist,* 1986, *26,* 398–404.

Davidson, S., and others. *The Children's Medicaid Program: Final Report.* Elk Grove, Ill.: American Academy of Pediatrics, 1988.

Department of Health and Human Services. *Toward a National Plan for the Chronically Mentally Ill.* Publication ADM 81-1077. Washington, D.C.: Department of Health and Human Services, 1981.

Docket, K. *Homelessness in the District of Columbia.* Washington, D.C.: Center for Applied Research and Urban Policy, University of the District of Columbia, 1986.

Franklin, J., and others. "An Evaluation of Case Management." *American Journal of Public Health,* 1987, 77 (6), 674–678.

Freund, D. *Medicaid Reform: Four Studies of Case Management.* Washington, D.C.: American Enterprise Institute, 1984.

Freund, D., and Hurley, R. "Managed Care in Medicaid: Selected Issues in Program Origins, Design and Research." *Annual Review of Public Health,* 1987, *8,* 137–163.

Freund, D., and Neuschler, E. "Overview of Medicaid Competition and Case Management Initiatives." *Health Care Financing Review,* 1986, annual supp., pp. 21–30.

Freund, D., and others. *Final Report: Medicaid Competition Demonstration Programs.* Research Triangle Park, N.C.: Research Triangle Institute, 1988.

Gersten, E. "Mental Health Issues of the Severely Disabled Psychiatric Client: Implications for Manpower Development and Staff Training." In M. Davis (ed.), *From Dependence to Independence: Staffing Community Programs for the Chronically Mentally Ill.* Boulder, Colo.: Interstate Commission for Higher Education, 1981.

Henderson, M., and Wallack, S. "Evaluating Case Management for Catastrophic Illness." *Business and Health,* Oct. 1987, pp. 7–11.

Hurley, R. E. "The Status of the Medicaid Competition Demonstrations." *Health Care Financing Review,* Winter 1986, pp. 65–75.

Hurley, R. E., Freund, D., and Taylor, D. "Emergency Room Use and Primary Care Case Management: Evidence from Four Medicaid Demonstration Programs." *American Journal of Public Health*, 1989, *79*, 843–846.

Intagliata, J. "Improving the Quality of Community Care for the Chronically Mentally Disabled: The Role of Case Management." *Schizophrenia Bulletin*, 1982, *8*, 655–674.

Knickman, J. "Case Management Services for AIDS Patients." Paper presented at the annual meeting of the Association for Health Services Research, San Francisco, June 1987.

Levine, I., and Fleming, M. *Human Resource Development: Issues in Case Management.* College Park, Md.: Center of Rehabilitation and Manpower Services, University of Maryland, 1986.

McCall, N., and others. *Evaluation of the Arizona Health Care Cost Containment Council.* Palo Alto, Calif.: Stanford Research Institute, 1988.

Mechanic, D. "The Challenge of Chronic Mental Illness: A Retrospective and Prospective View." *Hospital and Community Psychiatry*, 1986, *38* (9), 891–896.

Merrill, J. "Defining Case Management." *Business and Health*, July/Aug. 1985, pp. 5–9.

Mueller, J., and Hopp, M. "A Demonstration of the Cost Benefits of Case Management Services for Discharged Mental Patients." *Psychiatric Quarterly*, 1983, *55*, 17–24.

New York State Department of Health, Perinatal Unit. *Prenatal Care and Nutrition Program (PCAP).* Albany, N.Y.: Perinatal Unit, New York State Department of Health, 1988.

Perlman, B., Melnick, G., and Kentera, A. "Assessing the Effectiveness of a Case Management Program." *Hospital and Community Psychiatry*, 1985, *36*, 405–407.

Prottas, J., and Handler, E. "The Complexities of Managed Care: Operating a Voluntary System." *Journal of Health Politics, Policy and Law*, 1987, *12*, 253–269.

Rog, D., Andranovich, G., and Rosenblum, S. *Intensive Case Management for Persons Who Are Homeless and Mentally Ill.* Vol. 1: *General Findings.* Washington, D.C.: Cosmos Corp., 1987.

Schwartz, S., Goldman, H., and Churgin, S. "Case Management for the Chronically Mentally Ill: Models and Dimensions." *Hospital and Community Psychiatry*, 1982, *33* (12), 1006–1009.

Walker, G., and Weber, D. "A Transaction Cost Approach to Make-or-Buy Decisions." *Administrative Science Quarterly*, 1984, *29*, 373–391.

Wasylenki, D., and others. "Impact of a Case Manager Program on Psychiatric Aftercare." *Journal of Nervous and Mental Disease*, 1985, *173* (5), 303–308.

Williamson, O. E. *Markets and Hierarchies: Analysis and Antitrust Implications*. New York: Free Press, 1975.

————. "The Economics of Organization: The Transaction Cost Approach." *American Journal of Sociology*, 1981, *87* (3), 548–577.

————. *Economic Organization: Firms, Markets and Policy Control*. New York: New York University Press, 1986.

Wool, M., Guadagnoli, E., Thomas, M., and Mor, V. "Negotiating Concrete Needs: Short-Term Training for High-Risk Cancer Patients." *Health and Social Work*, 1989, *14* (3), 184–195.

Name Index

Subject Index